The Secrets Of Flexibility And Full Mobility

SADANAND PUJARI

Published by SADANAND PUJARI, 2024.

Table of Contents

Copyright

The Secrets Of Flexibility And Full Mobility

Unlock Your Body's Potential At Any Age With Just 30 Minutes A Day Using A Unique Method

First Edition: Jun 2024

Book Design by **SADANAND PUJARI**

About

You are only as young as your spine. This is the statement most often heard when discussing mobility and flexibility programs...and it's true!

This Stretching and Mobility Book is designed to help you improve your flexibility and increase your range of motion (mobility). By the end, you'll have been introduced to the concepts of stretching and mobility and better understand how they affect your posture, health, and daily functions. You'll also know the differences between static and dynamic stretching and learn how to perform stretches correctly.

Each exercise and mobility sequence builds on your flexibility, challenges your core strength, and improves your balance, movement efficiency, and strength.

In this Book, I'll even share simple and effective shoulder mobility exercises that will take just a few minutes out of your day but will help you get your shoulders moving and feeling the way they were meant to. Give yourself 5 minutes before or after a workout and notice your improvements. Your entire body will thank you!

Do you experience shoulder pain, tightness, or aches?

The good news is that shoulder pain can be easily overcome by focusing on the right exercises. Learning how to improve your shoulders' range of motion (mobility) and flexibility will open up an entirely new world of movement - and your whole body will thank you!

Intro and Key Concepts

Hi, everybody. It's a beginner's program in stretching, but even more so from people that are very inflexible, like myself. When I was a kid, when I was fifteen to twenty five, I was a black belt and I could stick my foot behind my head and I could do full splits and side splits and all kinds of impressive maneuvers. But between twenty five and now I'm fifty five. In the last 30 years I've done nothing but desk jobs, basically being a director or a therapist or a trainer. It's mostly sitting behind a desk. And here's what you have to do to ruin your stretch and become totally constricted. Whether you've stretched before or not, do absolutely nothing.

That's all you have to do. It's called atrophy, which is where things simply degenerate over time and constriction where things tighten over time. Now, I did the absolute worst thing like a human being can ever do. I sat at a desk. Let me demonstrate with a chair here why that's so awful. Basic care here, no trick photography, you sit in a chair. Here's what happens to damage your body. We said all you have to do is nothing and wait for the constriction. Now, if you want to get maximum constriction, make sure you don't extend any of your body parts. OK, when they're extended, they're elongated. And they would have a hard time constricting Y because they're extended. Now, how many of you sit at your desk like this? For those of you who still have a job, I'm assuming it's nobody.

OK, if you do it like that, your job will be the photographs. I'll get a great laugh out of it. Now show all my friends. But if you're doing a typical desk job, you've constricted your legs. So now these are going to tighten up and you can almost seem like they're seizing in place. Look, as I try to stretch my leg, I can't even get my legs straight out. That's terrible. OK, your arms will do the same thing. They start getting stiff in the shoulders, the neck, because you're holding it bad. Your arms are constricted. They're at an angle. They're not out like this. So they start getting tight in the biceps and across the shoulders and then up through the neck, especially as stress starts becoming a factor as well so maybe you're slouching in your chair a little bit. Now, your back is curved the wrong way and starts to tighten into place.

So bad posture, bent knees, bent arms is probably the least of it. But just hold this position for 10, 20, 30 years like I did, and you will seize up totally. That's all you have to do. It's not about old age. It's not about injuries. I thought I might have some medical problem or maybe in the martial arts I tore something, you know, or, you know, maybe I had some kind of degenerative joint disease or something. No, I just had moved very little. So I exercised when I worked out a little bit. But that had absolutely nothing to do with stress. So I looked like I was in decent shape, but I was totally inflexible. So now we're going to teach you how to break out of that. So here's the first concept that I want to give you in keeping with the constriction. I'll go ahead and I'll flash up on the screen. Maybe I'll put it up on the screen over here so you could see it.

This is fashion. Batia is tissue, the spider web-like tissue that forms over all the muscles. If I say cut open your leg right here and flip it back, you think you see, oh, nice red meat like you'd see on a steak. No you wouldn't. You'd see all that tissue on top. It surrounds every muscle. It's a fibrous material that holds things together. If you look at your garden hose reel closely, you think it's just this long green tube. Know what you're going to find if you look at it. There's this pattern, this hex pattern, like a checkerboard. It's got different fibers going through it to reinforce it. Otherwise, the pressure from the water would make it bulge and eventually rupture.

So to double or triple the strength of that hose, they make a net around it. So you've got this net around the outside of the tubing. That's the same thing, the same kind of netting. The fact that you have around your muscles to hold him in place, it's part of what helps them to work. But if you don't periodically stretch, which breaks up that fashion, that fashion will sit there, it'll thicken and it'll start to harden. It'll start to lose its elasticity and then we start to lose our elasticity. So a couple of things that you need to do. I'll do a bonus chapter at the end to kind of show you how to break up the fascia. You can literally massage it, grind it, use rollers, use different techniques to break up that . That's one way to do it in the second way is simply stretch.

You can almost see as you're stretching, you can feel the muscles pulling and you could almost feel the fashion going. Click, click, click, click, click. It's starting to break up. Why? Because you pulled it beyond its ability to stretch and it started to break up. So those are the two ways of literally grinding it, OK? Beating it down and stretching it out, so once you start to break that up, you start to get more flexibility. So the first thing that you're going to notice is not a great stretch at first, but you're going to notice that soreness starts to go away. I'm going to show you a great shoulder stretch that I do. And my shoulder pain used to keep me up, wake me up two or three times during the night and have to come out and use a massage roller. It was an automated one that was electronic and it had a kind of the shiatsu massage with the balls.

And I would wrap that around my neck and push it as hard as I could and it would just grind into those muscles. What was it doing releasing the tension of the muscles and breaking up the fashion. And that was the only thing that stopped the pain. But after just three days of doing this very simple stretching exercise with my shoulders gone and never, ever returning, even though I don't stretch that much anymore, I might do that stretch once a week or once a month. Doesn't matter because I broke up all that tissue and I trained my body not to tense that way anymore by what? Gently stretching it every once in a while. So I'm going to break down these chapters.

So we're doing just one, two, maybe three techniques, maybe four techniques. Sometimes we'll just do one thing to explain it. Well, I don't want it like one of these aerobic exercise chapters where they're jumping around and, hey, they show you something three or four times. And by about the fourth time you've got it on the fifth time they go into the next exercise. You may not have even got it yet. I want this slow and simple and broken down so you can see it, perform it with me or stop the tape, take some time, do it yourself. But I'm not going to be jumping on to the next thing. This is not an exercise chapter. This is a stretching chapter. I want you to get the technique. I don't want you to get a workout.

I'm here in basically dress slacks, in a polo shirt, and that's about what you need. As long as you can move around, you got some baggy pants and something you can move around your upper body. That's fine. You don't need a special workout outfit. We're not going to stretch that hard. We're not getting exercise clothes because we're not going to break a sweat. Very simple. Very delicate. Stretch it. Yeah, I've got two chairs. You can see them on either side of me. They're my favorite tool. Why? Because any time I need an assist, something's a little too much. I'm stretching over to the side and I go, oh, even that's too much weight. You can do a couple of things.

If you're doing a stretch like this, you can take your arm down and just go like this because now you're not putting this extra weight up above. You could put your hand on your hip to help ease things down or you could use the chair. So there's different stages. I want you to do gentle stretching. Hold the stretching. This is not something that builds up muscle. This is the build up. Stretch it and I don't want you to overdo it. So typical disclaimer, OK? I'm not a licensed physical therapist. I'm not a doctor, at least not that kind. Right. So check in with your doctor. This is not medical advice for educational purposes. If anything hurts, stop checking with your doctor first and the six other disclaimers I haven't thought of. OK, I'll put them at the beginning of the chapter.

But go gentle. Go easy, go slow. Now, the last thing I want to eat before I go in this beginning chapter is to go slow. The tortoise wins the race. If you're holding a stretch and you're doing about, say, maybe 60 percent of what you can do, that'll make sure you're not sore the next day. If you try to do 70, 80, 90 percent of what you could do, you may get a little more stretch and be very proud of yourself today, but then you're going to hurt your leg. And if you saw the next day and the next day and the next day, the next day, that's four days that you can't stretch. It's four days you're behind. You may have even injured the muscle. OK, so that'll be temporary. Some might be permanent. Who knows? Depends on how bad you did it. And you've lost your progress.

You've lost your momentum. It's going to start to seize up again. So slow and steady. This is a game of inches and millimeters, little, tiny bits every single day. Slow progress, even some plateaus. Once in a while, the first thing you want to do is get rid of the stiffness. Then we want to get a little bit of a stretch and then we're going to progress in our stretch. Then you can do the more advanced stretches and some other exercise chapter with the girl in the pretty leotard sticking her foot behind her head. If you want to go that far, that's great. But this is for people like me. So elderly people and flexible people, maybe even people who have injuries , really check in with your doctor and your physical therapist if you have injuries. Remember, this is just an educational chapter just for. This is not medical advice in any way, shape or form, but go ahead and join us and I'll see you in the very next chapter.

Warm Up - Understanding Static Stretching

Everybody, welcome back. Now, the first thing you want to do is rule number one, don't stretch cold muscles, cold muscles, tear warm muscles, stretch what I just said, cold muscles tear warm muscles stretch. So how can you warm up the muscles? Most relaxing way that I like to do it is I like to go for a nice walk. You want to get a little bit warmer in that. You can jog a little bit. I used to do some jumping jacks and I wanted to do something that was lower, impactful instead of doing the jumping jacks. I did the elliptical machine, very low impact, and I love the elliptical machine. But, boy, it really works the legs. I've also got a little recumbent bike, so I can do that as well. That's even gentler and easier than the elliptical machine.

But Of course, I can always set the tension. You can just do leg races. I just do the leg races that would warm it up or even lunge a little bit side to side. Anything that warms up the muscles. If you're going to be doing the upper body stretches and we do a few of those, then I would just lift some gentle hand weights or grab a half gallon of milk or something or some soup cans, whatever is a good weight for you and just move those to get the arms going. Now, once you've warmed up the upper and the lower body, you remember, whenever you warm up one part, you pretty much warm up the other one, because if if I were doing, say, squats with a weight, yeah, I'm working the heck out of my legs, but my whole body is hot.

Why is my forehead sweating? Because it goes through the entire body. Now, best to do a little bit of exercise that does work. The upper body does work, the lower body. But any exercise, even like I said, go for a walk, is going to have some effect across the body. So those are your basic warm up exercises. You can do any kind of warm up exercises that you like as long as it does a little bit of the upper body and more so on the lower body, because this is where you need to be doing probably 20 percent of your stretching and this is where you're going to be doing maybe 80 percent of your stretching.

Most people have problems with flexibility from the waist down, not from the waist up. So warm body stretches, cold body tears. Now, we also want to work the joints, warm up the joints, the insides of the joints, how do we do that? Just think about what joints you're going to be using and how they move. So a lot of times they'll start with neck rolls. We're back and forth with the neck, side to side with the neck, just move in any way you can think of that'll warm up the neck and start to stretch that out. That's actually a key area. A lot of people get stiff necks. Just doing that will give you a gentle stretch because it's hard to move it without stretching it a little bit because my neck is so stiff right now.

I was working out the other day. It's really stiff. Sometimes you just take a finger or two fingers and just move it over a little bit, roll the shoulders a little bit. So the neck is the first joint shoulders or the second joint. How can you move your shoulders? Shoulders basically move up and they move down. So this is a good warm up for it, right? They also move up and down in this direction, do them in that direction and they go round and round, do it in this direction, turn sideways and do it either or that's about all there is to a shoulder warm up. Now, the next thing is the spine in the hips. You turn to one side, you turn to the other, you turn to one side, you turn to the other.

You can lean back a little bit. You can lean forward a little bit. You can kick it out to one side a little bit. You can kick it out to the other side a little bit. You can roll it. That's about it, you just gently warm it up. Now, you can also hold on to something like the chair, you use the chairs quite a bit and just rotate the leg inside the hip. Great way to do it. Grab another chair. That's why I always like to. If you want to practice for balance, go one finger with the chair when you get better and your balance gets better, go like this. There are a lot of people who have balance issues that can help a lot to improve their balance and they don't need their cane anymore. OK, now.

The knees are the next joint. Think of it this way: how do I move the knee? I move it like this, OK? And it'll go a little bit sideways. So I basically just go like this a few times and I kick it out, kick it out straight from the side a little bit. That's it then. I'll go a little bit to one side, a little bit to the other and find your strength, and then what I do is I take my knees and I just roll them in this direction. Roll in this direction, pretty simple, pretty basic, and I'm kind of going up and down a little bit. That's it. Nothing too exciting. Sometimes I bend them in and bend them out. That's about it. Now you've warmed up the joints, now your body's ready to do the first stretches.

So let's do some real simple stretches just to get the body in the stretching move. So the first thing I do is I usually go off to one side and I go off to the other rather than to the other. Almost like I'm just warming up the hips again. But I'm trying to get a little bit of stretch. So let me grab onto something and I get just very gentle pressure, maybe like two fingers. He has to get a light stretch, you can use the chair again if you need to use that to kind of pull yourself around a little bit. Just two fingers. That's it. It's all a stretch you want. Then I want to stretch it side to side because that's where most people get stiff up.

Use the chair if you need to. So one way to do it is just over like this, but then you're putting all of this weight and all your body weight and nothing supporting. It's really going to pull here. If you want less weight, put one hand on the hip that will support it. And you can go over like this. If you want less weight than that, take the hand away. If you want less weight than that used to chair. See how you can always do injustice to your fitness level. Then just do the other side. And again, once you feel a light stretch, hold it, this is known as static, stretching doesn't bounce. There's a lot of controversy. Some people can bounce lightly if they do it very slowly and rhythmically, if they're very well stretched and they agree they can. I wouldn't lie because bouncin could hurt you.

Statik, stretch where you just come over and you hold it literally can't. I've never seen any scientific research where that hurt you. So the longer you hold any one of these stretches, the better off you're going to be. So that's your next strategy. Think of it this way. I'm already here. I already got the clothes on. I already got the chair out. I'm ready to exercise. I can hold this stretch for five seconds. One, two, three, four, five. Or I can go over and I can hold it for fifteen seconds. I'm only going to take ten seconds longer. It might extend, say, my fifteen minutes stretching routine into twenty minutes to double my stretching time, but I'll also double my results.

Let it be a little bit more than double. So why are there, especially if you're flexible, hold it for longer. This gives the muscles time to relax, to release. And what you're doing with stretching is your muscles could stretch, they could release if they wanted to weigh more than they do. Most people don't realize if the fastest is properly broken up. You could drop right now to a split. No problem. Why? Because a full split is a hundred percent of your range of motion. Your muscles actually have a hundred and twenty to one hundred and thirty percent range of motion. So you could actually put like two Boston phone books on either side and go all the way down to the floor in a full split or side split.

And that would be about one hundred and thirty percent. Why is it that I can only stretch about this far? OK, why? Because the muscles are not trained to do that, they tighten up. It's almost like if you were under hypnosis, you could do it. But your unconscious mind, because it's not trained to believe you can do the full split, it can't do it. So a lot of stretching is mental. So the longer you hold the static stretch and it says, hey, I can stretch at least this far and I know I can because every second I'm doing and I'm saying, hey, I'm doing it, I'm doing it, I'm doing it, I'm doing it. And then your body believes you can do what? You can do it.

And it says, OK, almost like a thermostat that you're slowly ticking up. He remembers the last setting and the next day you got another degree, another degree, another degree. So you do this in literally fractions of an inch of. Mm. A little bit more each day. That's how you are going to get all the way down a little bit of time each day and hold it to lock in those gains. So the longer you do it, the more you lock in the gains. So a lot of people, because they want to do it for long periods of time, they'll pick out maybe the twenty or so stretches that I'll show you. They'll pick five or six for their worst problem areas or the areas they just want to have a nice gain in.

And what they'll do is they'll do a simple stretch, you know, maybe like a hamstring stretch like this, but they'll do it while they're sitting on the couch. So their butts on the couch, they're sitting like this. They get into a position where they can feel some tension there. That's about 60 percent or 70 percent of what they can do for a stretch. And they hold it there. How long? A minute? Two minutes. Three minutes. Four minutes. I'll be leaving in five minutes, but usually between thirty seconds and three minutes is considered an elongated stretch that will really lock it in. Now, it is boring to sit going through all twenty stretches and hold it for three to five minutes each. That would be too long now to do it for ten or twenty or fifteen seconds, maybe even thirty seconds or a minute. That's not too bad.

You know, when you're doing say a dozen different stretches but three minutes times a dozen. Wow. You're up to what, almost forty five minutes. You know, you're out to like thirty five to forty minutes. That's a long time. It's so boring. But at night and you're sitting there and you're watching TV and you just get into the stretch and you hold it and I'm sitting here and watching TV. That's not boring at all. That's how you do it. That's the best way to do it. You do it the way that you like. Now let's do the next stretch. The next stretch is going to be a simple hamstring stretch. So literally the one I just showed you, put your leg out.

Now, interestingly enough, you can lock it in place like you see here. The knee is completely straight and then you want to just keep yourself alongside it. This is how bad my stretches are. That's plenty of tension for me, isn't that funny? Doesn't even look like I'm bending over. Here's me straight up, here's me stretching. That's how tight my legs are. I really need this. OK, now, I could bend over and hunch my back and make it look like I'm getting really close or do something like that. That's what most people don't know. Keep it nice and straight. Doesn't matter where you are. This is the before picture that's going to make the after picture so impressive.

It's OK. About 60 percent of what you can do, hold it now. If you're in as bad a shape as I am, I should probably hold it for about 30 seconds to a minute. If you really want to get the full benefit, like I said, do it while you're watching TV or something. Do it for three minutes and then go to the next leg. Now, interestingly enough, you can actually bend the leg a little bit and then go a little farther and you'll still feel it in the hamstrings. If you feel your leg right here, you can feel the hamstrings. And that's still a stretch. But your legs are not locked out. It's just two different styles of stretching, think of it this way.

One of the reasons I want to get more flexible is I thought it was embarrassing as a guy with a black belt and some food that I couldn't touch my toes. And I said, look, look, I can't touch my toes. It was a joke, so they said, well, you're doing it right, get a bend at the knee. So I bent at the knee and I said, Oh yeah, look, I can touch my toes. I guess it was a technique issue. Now, the funny thing is that's actually a stretch. You can go ahead and bend your knees and touch your toes and then kind of just pull the knees in a little bit, try to flex them out a little bit. And that's a stretch. Just go to where you get the stretch and you could stretch it like that or you can do it here.

And I would use the chair assist because remember, this isn't an exercise of putting your whole upper body weight and competing against your back muscles to see if you can tear them or not. It's to put the right amount of weight out in the right amount of stretch. So for hamstring stretches like this where you're trying to even do toe touches, I don't care what your level is, I would pretty much use the chair unless you're the expert level. So those are a couple of different hamstring stretches in the next chapter, we'll show you some more stretches to make it even more flexible.

Breathing - Stretching Secrets

Hey, welcome back, everybody. In a previous chapter, we were showing you how to do the hamstring stretches and we basically showed you how to do them here with the assistance of the chair. Put them out here, they can also do different levels. So what you should do is you should have something like the chair and let me grab my phone block. Now, what I'm going to do is instead of going here and maybe going into here stretching this far over, I'll go here, but not stretch as far here. So it's two different stretches. One of the lower levels, then a little higher than a little higher than a little higher. So there's two ways to stretch by leaning forward and creating tension here and by raising the leg slowly. I like to do a little bit of both.

They give you slightly different stretches. As you raise a little bit higher, it gets a little farther down on the hamstring. OK, more into the groin area. OK. And when you're here, it gets more down in this area towards the knee. So two different styles. You are a little bit different. Perfect. Blocks are great, these foam blocks are called yoga blocks, you can use them for different stretches, especially when you're really inflexible, but you're trying to get flexible. This is another aide, just like a chair. So say you were doing full splits, but you couldn't quite get down there to where you can put your palms down enough to be off the floor. Well, I can raise it by a block or I can turn this way and raise it even more.

Or I could put two yoga blocks out there, whatever I need, or go back to the chair. So these are just a nice little spacer to add those levels that you need to take the pressure off of the stretch or to slowly increase your stretch. These are like a six to eight dollar item on Amazon. So I would definitely get the yoga blocks. Now, the other stretch that you can do is from the side and you simply put your foot up here, you want to keep your toes pointing like I'm pointing towards you and all you want to do is just kind of go over. It's going to work the hips. It's going to stretch across the back. You tip your head and even get your neck a little bit. It'll work here. You'll feel it in here across the inside groin.

They call us the abductor's. And that works the inside of the leg, we just work the hamstrings, which are the backside of the leg. Now we're going to work the inside of the leg. Very simple. Again, if you need, help yourself with a chair. Putting the hand over the head can help. Sometimes that's too heavy. You put the hand on the hip, whatever adjustment you need to make. So I hope you're getting the theory more than the stretch is. A lot of these stretches are very common stretches that you may or may not need me to show you. It's the way in which we're doing the stretches that I want you to learn. Somebody's going to send me a comment.

So this was way too simple. Yes. Matter of fact, it's very hard to find complicated stretches even at the most advanced levels. You know, I saw one lady, she wrapped herself into the shape of a tulip. That was about the most advanced thing I'd ever seen. But she's a fitness expert and gymnast. You know, since the age of six, we're probably not going to get there. OK, now, one of the things that you can do is what's called active stretching. We said this was static stretching where you stretch a little bit and you just hold it. It's static. You're not moving. Dynamic stretching or moving, stretching is like this. I might do the same thing. I'm going to work the hamstrings, except instead of putting it up on the chair, here's what I'm going to do.

I'm going to swing the leg. This is on the upswing. Is pulling on the hamstring. This is a dynamic stretch, this warms the muscle works, the hips works, the muscles that support the stretch a little bit, which is good. A lot of people don't realize that a part of the reason why they can't stretch very well is for the muscle to stretch. It needs strength in the opposing muscle. So let me teach you a trick while I'm teaching you this theory. Say I'm trying to do this stretch and I want to improve my hamstring stretch underneath here. How do I do that? A, static, stretchy, B, dynamic stretching. See, by strengthening this.

So if I worked the quads. That's these top muscles here on your thigh, if I work those, then these muscles underneath will relax. Why? Because your muscles here are pulling against these muscles when these muscles are stronger than this one doesn't feel like it has to pull to support when these are weak, this will pull very tight to support the leg. So a trick that you can do in stretching is actually push down on the chair right now, pushing, pushing and pushing down the chair. If I push down about 50 percent as hard as I can push and I hold that for about 30 seconds, I will not only strengthen this muscle, the opposing one, which will help my stretch long term, I'm also fatiguing that muscle so that after the 30 seconds when I release it, my legs tired and it's easier to stretch. That's a great trick.

I know a guy who sold a kid on this, and that's all he did, he pushed out, pushed out, pushed out fatigue, that muscle, both by working it out and then holding it down for 30 seconds to 60 seconds and really wearing out that muscle, the opposing muscle, and then just stretching the opposite muscle, in this case, the hamstring. Fatigue, hold it for 30 seconds, push down, push down, push up, relax, breathe the outward breath, go down. Breathing is very important for stretching when you breathe in, your body gets energy when you breathe out, it releases energy when you breathe, then it takes in energy, which is tension. And when you breathe out, it releases energy, which is relaxation.

So a lot of people, you'll see them breathing as if stretching on the way down. I got a friend, you always see a little little person who looks so cute, looks so pretty when she does it and that's what she's doing. She does the bouncing thing. But every time she bounces, you see your little person, she goes. Where she knows she could touch her head to the floor, but that's what she's doing, even at her level. It's the breath and the relaxation. A lot of what's happening is you are tensing against you fighting it because you picture tense muscles as pain and we move away from pain. So when you're in pain, you tend to tighten up the muscle. If you tighten up the muscle, then it won't stretch. And if it's not stretching and it's not hurting, so your brain kind of plays a trick on you.

It tightens up so you won't pull forward. But your goal is to pull forward the fact that it's tightening, increases the pain, which makes you want to stretch even less and you get a terrible stretch. But by relaxing into the stretch and breathing into the stretch, you get past that mental trick of your body tightening up. It's tightening up to try to relieve you of pain, but it's actually causing the pain to things by tightening, you won't push forward. If I just push against you, you won't push towards me. And actually, that's what you're trying to do. So the trick is to relax, release and breathe. And then just hold wherever you're comfortable. That's it. OK. That's your lesson for this chapter, and I'll see you in the very next one. Take care.

The Secret Of Nerve Flossing (Part 1)

Everybody, welcome back, I'm going to show you another type of stretching. And again, these aren't necessarily unique stretches, although the next couple will be these are called neural or nerve flossing. I think nerve flossing is more accurate. So what you're doing is we talked about a static stretch. We talked about a dynamic moving stretch, and now we're looking at nerve flossing, which means kind of moving the tendon, moving the nerves. As opposed to pulling on them, so it's a different kind of dynamic stretch and what it does is it affects the nerves more so than the muscle tissue in the tents because the nerves are part of the equation as well. So think of it as just a different style of dynamic stretching.

And this will help you get gains that you otherwise wouldn't get. Almost all the stretches you see when you're taking a stretching chapter are about static stretching, static stretching and the occasional dynamic one which almost happens by mistake. So we've shown you how to do it properly. We've shown you the dynamic, how to do it properly. Now we're going to teach you a unique system called nerve flossing, which is moving stretches. OK, so first we need to do is all we have to do is we're going to get down on the floor and we're going to get our knees up to about a 90 degree angle. So straight here, straight here. And then we're going to point our toes or do those two legs.

And then all we're going to do is just rotate the legs a little bit. This gets and you can feel it gliding, you grab your hamstrings, that's why it's called nerf flossing. You can feel it. The hamstrings move at the same time they're pulling. Almost all the time, at least in the second half, from here to here, I'm getting a nice pull, but they're moving and sliding up and down. That's the flossing, just like you would do back and forth in your teeth. Simply going like this. You want to get a little support, you can hold it. And that's it, that's one Starliner Flosse. Now, reset the camera and I'll show you a second way to do it.

The Secret Of Nerve Flossing (Part 2)

OK, welcome back, everybody. Now I'm going to show you what must be the simplest form of nerve flossing ever created. It's a great stretch to show it to you right now. Simply sit up straight at your back up against the back of the chair. Put your leg out as straight as you can. You can see I can't get my way up here, so I'm going to go at an angle, but I'm able to lock out my leg. I couldn't do it there. I just simply move a little further in my chair. OK, I can hit it right about there. That's good. Now, all I'm going to do is point my toe out and point my toe in as I'm pulling in. This would be the breathing part. And if you felt back here once again, you could feel the tension sliding.

So you can feel this down in your calf. You could feel it all the way up the back of the leg into the hamstring. And that's all you do. It's nice and gentle and easy, that is. Nice, dynamic Nerf flossing stretch. Moving the tendons, moving the nerves and moving the muscle all at once you want, you can hold it for a couple of seconds up to you. On breathing during the tense phase. We then read that for you, then read that. That's it, so slim, so simple and just change be. Nice, gentle. Stretch, anybody can do it perfectly, so that's your very next strategy and I'll see you in the next chapter.

The Secret Of Nerve Flossing (Part 3)

Hey, everybody, welcome back, I love showing people how to do the nerve flossing. So here's another nerve flossing technique for you. Now everybody knows a typical hamstring stretch where you try to, you know, go down and touch your toes. We're going to do something similar, but we're going to do nerve flossing. We want the muscle, the tenants, the tissue and the nerves to flow back and forth. OK, so what we're going to do is we're going to bend at the knee a little bit, just put our heel into the ground, toes up, and then we're going to go.

But out, just up, just out. And we're just going to go up and down a little bit with our toes pointed, breathing on the downward stroke. And as you do this rocking motion, very gentle, very smooth, again, don't pull too tight. What you're doing is if you could see inside on the other side, you are just sliding everything back and forth in this area, so you're getting in the back of the calf, you're getting in the hamstring area, and it's just sliding gently back and forth as you drop down. As you rock, it is sliding back and forth.

That's why it's called nerve Flosse. Do that a few times, that'll get you a nice stretch all the way through here, and I'll tell you, I feel a little bit my quadrio feel a little bit in your knee again if you need to. You can hold yourself with a chair, but that's another style and nerve flossing. Again, feel your body, sense your body. You'll know if you're in the right position. You're doing it right because it'll feel right. You'll feel that nice, gentle glide, that nice, gentle stretch. Don't pull too much. Again, about 60 percent of what you can handle slow increments every day and you'll do fantastic. I'll see you in the next chapter.

Magic Of The Bear-Hug Stretch

Hey, welcome back, everybody. Now I want to teach you one of my favorite stretches in the introductory chapter. I talked a little bit about how I had shoulder pain. Oh, it would wake me up in the middle of the night. It was too much being hunched over a computer all day and just doing nothing for 30 years like we've talked about. It was just a lot of stress at work, too tight and tight and tight. And you're holding it in that position. Everything's kind of bunched up and held there under stress. Not good. So the shoulder pain got really bad until I learned a very simple stretch. I call it the bearhug stretch. All you do is you grab yourself like this and I want you to just go around in a circle, you lean to one side, and then you just start going in a circle very slowly like this and you will feel the stretch.

All the way across your back. Literally, from the tip of your scapula, this wing bone back here all the way down to your rear end, now your tailbone, and that will loosen all that up. And this is great because you're getting the entire back. You're breaking up all that farshid tissue and you get a nice stretch across your back if you have lower back pain, shoulder pain. This is a great one. So lean to one side. Roll it around. Oh, I feel so good. I usually get a nice stretch of either side at the end. And just shaking it out a little bit feels great. Let me show you that from the side. Same thing, give yourself a big hug, start at one side.

Just what your body can handle, I want you sensing your back. What's the right of my attention for you? If this is too heavy for you, again, just kind of keep you could almost go like this and support yourself with your arms doesn't work quite as well, but it takes the weight off, OK? Or you can lean back a little bit more and then go into it. And that would take some of the weight off as well. Bad posture, but that's OK. I feel so good, who knows, you can do it kind of one arm at a time, if you want to just go across, you could just pull it here a little bit. You go across and pull it here a little bit, but you don't get that nice wave across the shoulders.

I love this because I just get a wave of stretch heels just like a wave going across my back. And then I go the other way and another wave, all those tents, all those tendons and all that fashion, all that musculature all the way down the back, relaxing, releasing feels fantastic. That stretch alone should be worth what you paid for the Book. Like I said, it got rid of the muscular tension in my shoulders. It helped to alleviate the frozen shoulder issue that I had. It stopped me from waking up at night. It relieved a lot of pain for me to relieve a lot of pain for you. That's your tip for today. And I'll see you in the very next chapter.

Shoulder and Trapezius Stretch

Everybody, Now we're going to show you how to stretch out the shoulders again. How we're doing it is as important, if not more important, than the technique. You could jump on to YouTube and find all kinds of stretching chapters, but you're not going to find the science and the techniques that you're finding here. So one of the first things we want to do is think about how you stretch your shoulder to do a funny thing where I would show people hand techniques. It was how to grapple with people. And I call the technique doesn't go like that. So if you want to figure out how to grapple something, you start at the farthest extension, which is the fingers. And what I would do is I say, if you want to control somebody, just make their fingers go the way they don't go.

How can you control somebody then their thumb back like this? Because it doesn't go like this. See how they immediately have to move their entire body, then bend their fingers back like this and take all their fingers and bend it back like this, then take the thumb and take it and hyperextend the other way, don't go like that and start working your way up. The wrist doesn't go like that, doesn't go like that, and you can start manipulating people. So what you think about in the shoulder is which way does it move and which way do I get a stretch and then you'll be able to come up with your own stretches. So think of it this way. One of the things that we said the shoulder does is it goes up and down like this.

So one of the things that I want you to do is take a wall and literally just crawl your fingers up the wall to where you get a good stretch. When you get a good stretch, try to curl up a smidge more and maybe lean into it and lean away from it a little bit, lean into it and lean away from it a little bit, go up a little bit farther, feel the stretch, maybe get a little more stretch by dropping now while you're there and leaning towards the wall, that actually is the nicest stretch. Then once you get a little bit stretched out, see if you can go up a little bit further. Again, don't do more than 60 percent of what you figure you can do better to hold it for longer periods of time than to stretch it more. Remember that.

Better to hold it longer than to stretch it farther. I'd rather you want 60 percent of the way you could go and hold it for a minute. Then you went sixty five percent as far as you can go and held it for ten seconds or even held it for a minute, but then hurt yourself and put yourself back several days. Don't do that. So this is the first one which is going to give you this range of motion obviously. Yeah. Now the other way it goes is just across so you can pull your arm here or you can put your arm across something and then just turn into it, gently turn into it, just hold it lock. Put your hand there if you need to and just move into it very gently again. You can hold it or you can do it dynamic where I'm just very gently moving back and forth. Don't bounce like one of these.

Don't bounce like that, but a smooth roll that you can do a smooth roll. That you can do, but I tend to just stretch it, hold it, wait, hold it, release, shake it out, move it around, do it a little bit more. Then go to the next stretch now, as you're doing this one, you've actually got different angles of stretch. This is where it becomes unique. So you do it here and you do it here and you do it here, then you do it here, then you do it here. Same exact motion. Different levels. It's going down through and then I'm going to go below where I started and turn it. You know, as you go really low, you have to get a little closer to the wall, right? That works at every possible angle within this range. So now we did it this way and now we did it across the body at all the different angles that starts activating different stretches, different muscles. You'll feel it.

People go like this and they say, oh, I stretched it across here. Now I'm done. Now I usually go like, one, two, three, four, five. So middle to above to below. That gives me five different stretches. That's usually plenty. But I've seen people in about an inch at a time. They really like to refine it, get a hell of a stretch if you do it like that. OK, now next stretch, your arm goes up and it goes over, so. What you can do is just simply grab your elbow and give it a light stretch. Some people will use a resistance band where they'll grab on to the resistance band and then they'll pull it back here. You can do that.

That's a little bit more advanced. OK, normally, even just sometimes, the weight of your arm is enough like that. Or just, again, a couple of fingers very gently. And again, you could even move it out and in a slightly different stretch, depending upon how you are doing it out here? Way in here. A little bit different. OK. Now, that's pushing it about as far this way as it goes, how about if we go as far this way as it goes? Well, the easiest way to do it is to start with something that has levels. I like this because it has levels, but you can use a short chair, you know, or a coffee table or say, your dining room table. Then you could use maybe the back of a chair. Then you could use the top of your couch. Whatever you have, you'll get creative, you'll find things.

I just use my entertainment center. So I will start with this one. And if I want to get a stretch, all I do is I go down a little bit, get the stretch when I get stretched out, if I can go to the next level and I do go down a little bit more. OK. Here's another legitimate cheat. Remember our old friend, the yoga block says I've only got one level. Great. Put that there. Put the yoga block there. Now, I have gained a little more height. I can flip the yoga block up now. I still got a little more height. At one level become three, it's like the loaves and fishes I got in my yoga block, so the yoga block is a great strategy to give you small increments literally of about two to four inches at a time. So this is about four inches here. This is about six inches here. And that's why I say about two to four inches. Perfect.

Matter of fact, if you want to think about it, I think it's eight inches across. So you could go like four, six and then eight. It's a little less dirty when you do it that way, though. OK. Now, one of the things that I like to do to warm up the shoulders is do something that's called dynamic tension. This is the old classic Charles Atlas. The guy comes in, kicks sand in your face at the beach. OK, what he would do is he would take one muscle against the other and just strain it so you could do one muscle against the other. You can really feel that in the shoulders I'm pulling with one. Against the other, I could also push with one against the other. This is a nice warm up great to warm up the muscles before you stretch. Remember, warm muscles stretch, cold muscles tear.

You can also do this with nothing I can push this way, and I have pushed this way, this is muscle against muscle within the arm. I'm just kind of imagining a weight there. But I'm actually tensing one muscle against the other. So you can really see it in the triceps there. When I do it, the triceps activate. So if you're doing a curl. Same thing now you're warming up the arm, one muscle against the other, you're doing an overhead, too, like you're lifting a weight over your head. Bull activates all the shoulders, warms them up. OK, so warm up, stretch and relax and breathe. Just stretch. Now, you also want to go across the body. We talked about doing it like this.

You can also use a tool for that. I usually just put my hand on the wall and I twist into it this way and I put my hand against the wall and I twist into it this way. Well, I'll tell you, that's about every stretch you ever need to work all the shoulders we taught you. The bear hug stretches to get from the shoulders on down. So now you've done the entire area, the shoulder all the way around the other muscle that you need to get is in here, you get that mostly with the bare stretch. They can also do that just by pulling down here and pulling down here. You also feel that right across here. This one is the trapezius, it's called, it's just this muscle here, his whole shoulder muscle up here, the upper shoulder muscle as opposed to the lower shoulder muscle, just good massage is the best way to loosen that up.

There's no real way to really stretch that muscle. That muscle is most likely to release if you exercise it and fatigue it. The way to do that is all those muscles do is they move your shoulders up and down. So you know what the exercise for that is would be shoulders up, move your shoulders down, move your shoulders up, move your shoulders down. A lot of times if you do it with a sigh, bring them up, tighten the tension release, bring them up quick drop, bring them up, quick drop in and exhale. Like you're saying, that's the best way to release the trapezius muscles. That's your tip for today. And I'll see you in the next chapter.

Groin Stretch - Inner Thigh

Hey, welcome back, everybody. Now I want to show you some side stretch ones. This would kind of be a lead up to doing side splits, but I don't think we'll even get that far. It's not that kind of a chapter, but I do want you to be able to work the inner groin muscles a little bit, because that's about the only one that we've only done a little bit of work on to strengthen the legs a little bit and to get a stretch. Hope you can see this with it, with a chair in the way. I'm basically putting my hands on the chair and all I do. And this is why I got socks on a slippery floor. It's just letting that leg go out until it locks. And I'm bending this knee and just getting a little bit of stretch right in here in the groin area, very like, very gentle, just what it can handle. And then you hold it for a few seconds, you let it back in.

If you want to do a flossing exercise, you can do a smooth in and out, just like you just rubbing the floor with your foot, even the floor, a little massage with your foot. That's it. Then you switch sides. Then you can hold it. When you have more time, I don't want to, you know, demonstrate a three minute hold or 30 second hold. Hold it, breathe out, and that's as much or as little as you can do. That'll give you a good strength in the quads, which we said will help you work the opposite side. It's going to give you a good stretch on the abductor's. So perfect, perfect stretch. Very well supported. Make sure you don't slip. Make sure you got a good, sturdy chair. That's all you need to do this stretch. Take care.

Benefits Of Yoga Stretching

Hey, everybody, welcome back, Now I'm going to show you a little bit of yoga, just the simplest of yoga. Now, what is yoga? Yoga is just simply the stretching of the muscles. It's what they call studio yoga. There's two kinds of yoga. Yoga is where you're going to a higher mental level. That's one form of yoga other than studio yoga, which is all about the stretching and the positions versus the spiritual aspect. So we're going to be looking at the stretching and the positions, not the spiritual aspect. It is a totally different chapter. So I want to show you that it's not this weird, ancient mystical art. It's simply a movement in stretching. And that's what we're going to do.

We're going to do the simplest yoga stretches known to man. And anybody can do all I can do. You can do it. So the first one we're going to do is simply the cat stretch. So you get in this position here and then arch your back up. And bring your head forward and arch it in. Arch it out, stretching especially the lower back. And then down. Out. How? That now, if you want, in any position. You can just kind of work it around a little bit, move your hips, move your shoulders, loosen stuff up. I like to extend it out and then wiggle it, because that gives me a good stretch of my shoulders and my back. You can even go back and forth like this. This is actually called child pose.

They just go down here and they stretch across the back. So that's the second pose. Feels really good. And that's all you do. Nice and gentle. Work it, he shifts like this a little bit, you get a little bit more stretch, this is just a rolling technique. Perfect.

But back to here. Now they've got a position where you go sweeping through and they do a downward dog. All I do is I get my butt down to the mat and I'm just going to lie down like I'm taking a nap for the day. I'm going to put my hands by my side and I'm going to see how much is usually right around where your face and your shoulder is. I'm just going to push and see if I get a little curve on my back just to flex the back a little bit. A little stretching in the back. You can even put your elbows down.

This is what I do when I want to hold it. Just get in a stretch in the back and then I do the rolling technique. This loosens up stuff in the back, in the hips. You move your shoulders, he loosens things up in the shoulders. All I'm doing, whatever level you can get to, you can't go that high. Then you go here. I mean, you can do it a lot of different ways. You can just do it here. I mean, you can set any level you want. You could use the yoga blocks on my back that are very stiff. I had several back injuries. This is about what I can do. So imagine if you're, you know, 50 like me and even 60 or 70 or 80, if you had no back injury, you could probably do this. That's it. So.

That's one stretch. This is two stretches. That's the cat stretching the child's pose. Nice pull on the back. From here, a lot of people just go in different directions. Sometimes a nice hand movement is good. Just like you walking around. Stretch here. Stretch here. Put your hand here and a hand here, turn a little bit this way. Hand here, hand here, wherever you can get, you can't, you know, grab the mat, whatever you got to do, wherever you can grab it, just a gentle stretch in this way. Stretch to this side. Stretch to this side. Stretch to this side, stretch to this side, get down and go around. If you do that, you'll have wonderful flexibility all around the middle area, which is the spine, that's the area that tends to get the most type even though it's a good stretch.

Just moving it around. Do you like figure eights with your shoulders? Anything you can do that you feel loosens it up. You're doing it right. Just move it in different ways where it's tight for you, send your body, listen to your body, go slow, take your time, make sure you warm up first of all the things that we've been teaching you. But see how those poses are so simple. They're not complicated, but they do a huge amount of what the remaining poses do, especially for what you need. If you're not going to be a yoga instructor, you're not a professional athlete, you're not going to be Superman jumping over tall buildings. You don't need this for any particular reason except you want better health and you want to be able to move well as a normal human being and not be in pain, not have tension, not have the infirmities of old age.

You just want to be fluid and healthy and alive. And this is plenty what I've shown you everything above that is for some kind of specific task, athletic performance or maybe a job requirement. You do a lot of heavy lifting and you need, you know, more stretching and strength around your back or in your legs or something like that. But otherwise, a lot of exercises that they show you on the Web, on the Internet and in the gyms and things like this, they actually have nothing to do with what a human being is going to do during the Book of their day. They serve no other function than building up muscle for, I don't know, for vanity, for parents and just something to do when you're at the gym. That's your tip for today. That's your new strategy. Your new technique that's going to help create a new you. Thanks so much.

Tools To Release Fascia & Tension

Hi, everybody. I know you may have just seen me seconds ago, but for me it's been about an hour and a half. Why? I've been trying to find a few simple tools that I wanted to share with you today, but my wife hit him. Now, if you ever come up with a chapter of how to get wise to stop hiding things in the house from their husband, I'll buy your training Book. Now, the first thing is a roller bar. There's actually a technique called Galusha. I always mispronounce it, but it's basically breaking up that Farshid tissue by using tools to dig in and they really dig it. It's called scraping. Why? Because they take the tools and they scrape against the skin and the muscles and it turns beet red.

You will bruise. There's some blood vessels that may get broken underneath. I mean, they're really grinding in to break that fashion, to break it up around the muscle. For some people have really set in tissue in their muscles. They just need to really get in there and grind it. Now, there's some massage therapists that'll do facial release and that's what they're doing. If you've ever had a deep tissue massage, just multiply that by five. And that's what it takes to break up that fashion. And they'll do it by stretching, pulling, tearing at it, rolling it back and forth between their fingers, basically, any way they can really dig in there and break it apart.

Now, the other way to do it very gently, it won't be as invasive and it won't be as intense and it won't be as thorough. But you can do it through something called rolling. Now, rolling can be done a couple different ways. I've got a couple of different tools here for you. I've got a classic foam roller and what people will do with this is they'll simply put their weight against it, like lie on the floor and then they roll back and forth on the floor and let it hit the different areas. You do the front. You do the back, you do the side. You could do your shoulders. You can do your arms. You could do it inside. You can go outside.

You could cross the middle of your back. You can roll it. But rolling is simply putting pressure with your body, any body part against the roller and then going back and forth. And that just crushes them and helps to break it up. Some people even roll a little bit this way, as opposed to just like this, so when they have their leg on it, they'll roll their leg across it a little bit. And a lot of times what people will do is they'll really work on or even hold and grind it to and apply extra pressure to certain areas that are really tight to create a release. So some people will do this before stretching or working out. Some people will do it after stretching or working out.

So it helps for stretching, helps for faster release, and it also helps to release some tense blocked areas. That's kind of an old massage technique. You can massage something by manipulating it and moving it. You can massage something by stretching it as technique number two, and the third one is just apply pressure and don't let it off. That's kind of what the rolling is doing. It's putting pressure on. And if you have a really bad spot, you just hold that spot. It keeps the weight and the pressure on it in the muscle fatigues and eventually has to release. You can't hold it any longer. So that's the classic foam rolling. Then there's roller bars. This is part of the Maokai.

They will have the rollers in. All you do is roll it along the muscle. I love it along the upper calf muscles here. The quads, they call them. Oh, that feels good. If you want to get the hamstrings, you go underneath. Sometimes it's good to do it like this. Sometimes it's good to do it lying down, getting behind the calves on the sides of the calves. Great for doing the legs, harder for doing the arms, because you don't have your two arms to push down with. You have to have somebody do that for you. But for things like the forearms, I can do pretty well. If I've been working at the gym, I can do it for the biceps. It's actually not bad. If you need a little added pressure, just push against something like a wall and use that to kind of hold one side.

You know, it's got to be a well, you know, like much as you're probably going to scrape it, do it out in the garage or something like that or on the side of the house. So this type of rolling is great. When my wife does it, she can get my whole back. That's really nice. Great. And then again, this is like an eight, nine, ten dollar Amazon item. I got a kit with a three piece kit. It's got this ball and it's also got the peanut peanut two balls stuck together, which is good for getting like the arms or the small, the back hitting both sides it wants for rolling. And then the main roll was like a fifteen dollar item. So maybe I got twenty five dollars here.

Boom. Here's another great one. This is like a fifty cent item. Tennis ball, tennis ball. You could take in a roll on an area, but you're not going to get a lot of pressure. But sometimes you can just bang it with a tennis ball and that'll release the muscles and break up the fashion a little bit so you can do some tapping. I call it basically pounding on your leg or pounding on an area. You can do that. But the classic technique is you take something like a chair when I get a fresh chair here. Lip locks need a hardship. This is a padded chair, but I'm just going to show you the basic concept of it. All you do is you take the ball and you put it underneath your leg and then just let it sit there and put pressure on it. You can go up and down. You can let it sit there for a while.

That's going to create a release. But the best thing is to be able to roll back and forth, maybe over a six inch area, three inches forward, three inches back, and that will grind in almost like the nerve flossing and start to release the fashion, then move it forward a little bit to the next spot until you get the entire length of your leg perfect. If you can get your leg high enough up that you get a table, you can also do the calf as well. So that's a great way to break up those hamstrings, just using the tennis ball. Now, another great way to do it. You would be surprised how much of the tension in your legs, in your hamstrings.

You know, part of the reason why you can't touch your toes and you have so much flexibility through your legs is actually your feet. So what you need to do is get a tennis ball and on a hard surface, you could do it in a car. But if your carpet's not too thick and there's not too much pad, but on a hard surface, maybe tile floor linoleum, simply put the ball down and just start rolling it and put it at any spot in your foot that feels good and then apply some pressure and hold it, hold it, hold it. Like it doesn't hurt. You're doing it right. You feel some tension there. That's probably where you need it. Then move it to another spot and just push down on that. Leave it there for a few seconds, just as if you were doing a stretch. Do it again in another spot.

And what you're going to find is you're going to break up the fashion, the foot. You're going to release a lot of tendons and tension. A lot of mental tension is stored in your feet, if you like, acupressure in those types of things. Reflexology, there's a lot of those points on your foot. Some people do this with a spiky ball. They don't do it as hard. But the spiky ball will actually stimulate all those acupressure reflexology points. But this is really just to get that release. And if you're a person that's on their feet all day, this can feel fantastic.

So you can do it as light or as hard as you want. Again, listen to your body, do it very lightly the first time, then go a little harder, a little higher, a little harder. See how your feet and your body respond. But you may find you've got a lot more flexibility from the waist down simply because you use this ball.

Extra Stretching Fitness Resources

Hi, everybody, I made this for people like myself that had difficulty stretching. Now, this was originally going to be an hour long training. We obviously want a little bit over that, but I always love to give you the extra. So I'm doing this bonus chapter for you to give you still more. I want you to be able to continue learning even after this training is long gone. So keep going back to it as a resource. But I've got additional resources for you because obviously I couldn't teach you every stretch that's out there or this would be a twenty six week Book.

So I'm going to give you some additional resources, places where you can go to continue your education. Let's look at some of the first ones. Now, the first one is Bohle Beautiful. I love this because they use beach shots and gorgeous scenery. Now, this is the pretty girl in the leotard that I told you not to watch. But she does a great job of going through all the stretches from a yoga perspective, but does virtually every stretch under the sun. Now, obviously, I'm going to trust your intelligence. You need to adjust this to your level. But she goes slow. She describes it, she explains it, tells you what you should do, what you shouldn't do.

So in that way, it's perfect training. Check it out. I think you really like it. Now, the next one is called Rehab My Patient. So these are done by physical therapy experts. They're broken down to segments. A lot of you who are a little bit older, like myself or maybe even older than myself into your senior years or maybe even younger than myself. But you've had some difficulties that have caused some of these stretching issues or you just happen to have these difficulties. These are ways that you can go through and learn some physical therapy elements to help deal with different areas.

And they also have some stretching chapters as well to continue our theme. I just want to make sure that kind of on every level you're taking care of. Now, guerrillazen fitness. This is a little bit of a 50-50 split, I imagine if you're trying to improve yourself, improve your body, you might want to do a little bit of strength training as well. So this has stretching and fitness chapters, but it also has some weight lifting and strength building chapters. Perfect for you, if that's what you're looking for. Now, we've also got yoga with Bird. There's a lot of different people that teach yoga, just like Bojo fitness. But I think she does a really good job, doesn't she? Nice and slow against the pretty girl in the leotard.

But she's a very well trained fitness instructor, and explains the importance of everything. Walk you through it, it is nice and slow. Of course, you can always pause the chapters or go back over them. But I just think that she does a really nice job and is very comprehensive. So if you have a specific area you want to work on, she'll have a chapter for that. Now, some of this is also going to incorporate some fitness type stuff, too, to not only stretch the muscles, but to strengthen them. And that should be perfect for you. Now, if you're looking to get a little bit more fit and you're my age, I'm fifty five or maybe younger than me. This is called Mad Fit.

This will take you through and show you all kinds of different great exercises and fitness things that you can do with little or no equipment, which is fantastic. So. Great fitness chapters, this will give you the strength as well as the stretch and remember, strength supports stretching. Now, if you're my age or a little bit older, we've got ones called Senior Fitness with Meredith. I like these because she's constantly adding new content. She takes it slow. She walks you through each exercise. She does it with minimal equipment, just a few pieces of equipment that you can buy on Amazon or no equipment.

So you might have an investment, maybe seventy five dollars if you bought every piece of equipment she shows there, certainly no more than one hundred dollars and she respects you. So she understands that if you're doing senior fitness, you might be everywhere from wheelchair bound to fairly athletic for your age. Perfect. So she respects it at all levels and at whatever level you're at, you're able to adapt these fitness routines that she's doing to match your level. Absolutely perfect. Now, a lot of people ask me, how often should I stretch and we really didn't address this in the chapters, so how often should you stretch? I stretch every single day.

Now, why do I do that? Probably about every other day. I'm doing a very light stretch, which means just enough to elongate the muscles and alleviate any stiffness that I have. I'm really just gently loosening up the body. You should do that every day so that that fashion doesn't set in place, so that your muscles get used to being alongside it, but you're not straining them on a daily basis. So that's your light day on the heavy day, maybe every other day or every third day. It's up to you. Go ahead and do the heavier stretching where you're trying to make some gains and you stretch a little bit at a time. Remember, don't overdo it. One day of overdoing it is going to wipe out at least a week's worth of gains.

So slow, gentle, easy and steady wins the race, so one day, like one day for a game, one day like one day, four games perfect. And, Of course, stretch and limber up before you do any type of fitness routine, remember, warm the muscles before you stretch your muscles, stretch cold muscles, tear. Don't forget. OK, those are your bonus tips and bonus resources, everybody, thanks so much. I really appreciate it. These will show you all my other health fitness resources. I teach in three basic areas.

Our old motto was healthy, wealthy and wise. So I teach psychology and self-help personal development type stuff. I teach business and career development, money making type stuff, and I also teach fitness. We literally do want to make you healthy, wealthy and why. So if you enjoy these chapters, we have chapters that can help you in virtually every area of your life. That's why I created that model. Advanced Ideas, Making You Healthy, wealthy and what we want to hit the three major areas, your life, health, wealth and wisdom. Thank you so much. You've been fantastic. And I'll see you in my very next training. Enjoy your bonuses.

Introduction To Functional Fitness Training

When you say the word health, you are referring to the well-being of yourself or others, so naturally, health becomes a personal matter, especially when it revolves around your own health. Everyone wants to be in better health, which is, again, a very natural impulse. The first and easiest thing you can do to better your health is to eat properly and work out routinely. Eating properly can become dieting and monitoring what comes into your kitchen. Working out, on the other hand, can be somewhat trickier. Working out doesn't have to mean you aim to become a bodybuilder or weightlifter, though those are possible achievements to gain from working out. It could simply mean you want to maintain a certain weight or keep your body moving properly and functionally in such cases to maintain proper health. You don't need dumbbells and treadmills, only a functional fitness routine.

What Is Functional Fitness

In this chapter, we'll talk about what functional fitness is, functional fitness defined. You may not have heard the term functional fitness before reading this, but the truth is that functional fitness is all around you. Functional fitness refers to a type of fitness where you keep your body moving in simulated routines that resemble everyday tasks. Now, most people imagine working out as this fantastical imagery where you have a solid core and large protruding biceps that bulge every time you lift weights. This image is one that's better to burn. Not everyone can live this fantasy, and in most cases it's unrealistic and impractical. You can't be your average person when you look like Dwayne Johnson. And honestly, keeping such a physical shape is harder to do than maintaining a normal one.

It'll become an extra weight on your shoulders that you'll quickly get tired of carrying. An easier and more reasonable way to maintain a fit figure is by sticking to simpler goals. What most people want is to be able to perform with the most practicality on a daily basis to ensure they drop the weights and stick to more natural movements. This is where you resort to functional fitness. With functional fitness, you'll be doing squats, lunges, stretches and pumps that are closer to home. All of these movements will resemble or become more exaggerated versions of actions you do every day.

Take lunges as an example, lunges are the movement of stretching out and bending your leg, though you'll never be found walking in this cycle, it's imitating the movements you make in more extreme cases, going up the stairs and running use the same actions as walking does, but with more strength and power. By doing lunges, your muscles and joints become accustomed to the strong pull and strain and therefore perform more effectively as you run. As you grow older, you may have found that your body can't do the same things it used to. It's all right since this happens to everybody. Unfortunately, the more lethargic you become, the faster this will happen to you. So it's better to get up and get moving in any way that you can.

Functional fitness can be performed anywhere at any level of difficulties. For instance, you can even use your own body weight to perform the exercises without using any gym equipment. As long as you're moving in a way that can benefit your body, you're doing some kind of functional fitness. It's better than lifting the heaviest weights and then snapping when you're trying to load groceries into your car, complimenting functional fitness with your lifestyle. As mentioned earlier, hoping for the perfect ten out of ten body is unrealistic and quite impractical. The basic aim should always be maintaining a healthy body. You as a person are satisfied with it. Being fit is only a further benefit to yourself. That said, your exercises shouldn't interrupt your schedule, but rather flow inside of it.

Once it becomes a problem. To find time for your workout, a red flag should signal in your mind. Here's some tips to keep in mind when crafting a workout routine that works for you. Firstly, it shouldn't take long at all. A fifteen to twenty five minute routine is enough to make a difference. As long as you're implementing this workout every day, you don't need anything that hard, just simple, repetitive movements to properly pump your muscles. These few spare minutes can be early in the morning or after your busy day. Typically it's better to work out before you start your day's work. Otherwise doing anything at the end of the day will tire you out more than you'd usually be. You can also develop intense strain and pain if you remain idle for too long after a workout.

Another idea is to spread out your workouts through the week on days, your working workout for only fifteen minutes and on weekends or holidays workout for twenty to twenty five minutes. This way you won't tire yourself out when you have other things to do. Any system that suits your schedule is fine, so long as you're getting the essential minimum of 15 minutes. When you start out, keep all of your moves minimalistic, nothing too extravagant. That'll pull your muscles before you've even used them. No weights in the beginning. They will strain your muscles far too quickly. Once you're used to the burn from simpler workouts, you can apply small two or three pound weights and never start out big. It's unhealthy, unrealistic and impractical.

When you're working out, keep some water nearby and wear active wear. Always keep yourself hydrated when working out. Even if you don't feel tired while working out. There's always an after effect. Have lots of free space around you with a clean carpeted floor, or purchase yourself a yoga mat for moves where you bend or lie down. The more space you have, the fewer chances there are of an injury or breaking something near you. Is functional fitness right for you? Not everyone is capable of working out, though society has now made it something very normal. You may not fit in with this group of people that can work themselves to the bone. If you're baffled, bear through for there is an explanation.

Yes, it's true that functional fitness basically tries to cover all generic movements, reinforce your stamina, strength and range of motion. Yet still, what about those people who can perform daily tasks and nothing more than illnesses, weakness, age and injury can prevent you from doing more than what you're currently capable of, though you may feel you're ready for more. Your body may not be remembered before anything else. There's no need to push limits that shouldn't be pushed. In typical cases, functional fitness can cover most people's necessities. Whether you're hunting for a better body or a more productive day. Functional fitness reaps the benefits to age you down that road.

But for those with physical restraints and disabilities, there's no harm in realizing what you're not capable of doing. If you're injured, then it's a momentary. Unless the after effect is lifelong, a scrape or bruise will put you down for a few days. Broken bones will keep you grounded for a much longer period and in some severe cases the rest of your life. If bodily functions are really something you wish to improve, though, then there's no reason for you to carelessly carry yourself around. Injuring your limbs or other monetary obstacles can be surgery, pregnancy, traveling or moving and other impactful events in life.

There's no way you can keep up working out each and every day, especially if you have other things on your agenda to attend to. Not if you miss a day. Simply get back into the routine as soon as you can. The longer you wait, the harder it will be to return to your former glory. As you grow older, you'll become more limited to what you can do. Bone health and newly developed issues have to be taken into account before you attempt any kind of workout. The older you become, the less likely it'll be that you can fit functional fitness into your habitual routine. That's why it's always better to start such things in your best health when you have no obstacles.

Some people are born with permanent issues that prevent them from working in certain positions. There are many situations you may find yourself in. Being born with weaker bone strength could mean you're incapable of working yourself past a certain degree. So the basic idea here is that demotivation is the countering effect of motivation. It's a block that prevents you from becoming motivated and insecure . If anything, motivation, breathing or digestive issues can also hold you down from working out since these areas will be directly affected.

Benefits Of Functional Fitness

In this chapter, we'll learn about the benefits of functional fitness. There are multiple benefits to functional fitness that can easily become part of your daily routine to convince you further of the powerful impact functional fitness can have on your life. Here are some benefits that functional fitness can provide you with easier movement. It's basic knowledge that the more you move, the easier it becomes to move later on in life. Remember those days as an infant when you were clambering onto furniture trying to figure out how to walk? Of course not, since you were, after all, an infant.

But it's a perfect example for this point. As an infant, you'd always have fallen over, cried a little, and then returned to your attempts to get up and walk. The more you did it, the better you got at doing it. Since your body steadily adjusted to the actions, the same procedure occurs when you're working out. The more you repeat these actions, the more accustomed your body gets to them and the easier they become to perform. Once your body is used to these movements, running, bending down, jumping and heaving will all become a lot easier. That's why I'm making functional fitness. A daily part of your routine is so important. If you lose the momentum of working out regularly, you'll also lose the stability and consistency of your movements and you may even get sore much quicker than you might have before.

The best part about functional fitness is that you can start anywhere with it. There's no grand expectation to meet or deadlines to pay up monthly subscription fees, just your own personal made goals and free time. Functional fitness, and its most basic to most intense form will always remain a low impact workout. This means beginners can commence at an easy pace without the worry of working out to be too hard on their body. On the other hand, those who already have it implemented in their schedule will easily be able to pick up their pace without leaving their comfort zone. Once you've gotten down the pattern of your functional fitness routine and you have a clear idea of what you're capable of, keeping yourself fit will never be easier.

Movements are always done best in a flow. Without a system to your movements, you'll end up fumbling and tumbling in everything you do. Practice makes perfect and this applies to everything, even the way you walk. The more you do something, the more progress you'll endure to succumb to the best of your ability. So for the best performance each day with fast and steady movements, functional fitness is the best solution to making your body perfectly functional. Stronger support and immune system, though you may not realize it immediately when you work out, your body becomes stronger. It's more resistant to attacks upon it.

Now, when saying attack, this doesn't refer to life threatening events, only simple accidents that can harm your body. Scratches and bruises will have less effect on your body if you work out on the daily. Instead of having a throbbing bruise on your knee for days on end, it may hurt for a few hours and then feel like an irritating itch. You'll also be able to handle more impact on your muscles while you're on the move. If running and going up the stairs were an issue before working out can help you make those issues disappear. Functional fitness is the best kind of workout for improving your daily functional movements. Since this is the primary focal point in all the exercises. With each workout, you'll also feel a surge of adrenaline run through your veins, which is a good thing.

Adrenaline gives you extra power and more stamina when you need it. Adrenaline will be provided to you at a faster rate than if you didn't work out along with the buildup of adrenaline. There's also a buildup of stamina. With this, you'll be able to perform for longer periods of time and do more than you can usually do. If heaving the groceries tired you out before then. After proper functional fitness, you'll be heaving more than bags with ease in no time. Every day will be so much easier to conquer. When your body is stronger and sturdier. You'll also feel more energized and confident the more your body can handle.

Functional fitness can help you increase your general health in everyday life. Functional fitness can also open more doors for you. You can try new sports or hobbies that involve going out with clearer certainty. With a newer, fitter you, there is more you can do, more options you can discover. Stamina and strength aren't things you can develop overnight, but once you have them, all of your days will change for the better. Walking to work will seem less of a hassle. Running in the evening will appear to be more fun than irritating, though you'll never be able to compete with the heavy bodybuilders out there by only doing functional fitness. You can reach full potential in more material events in life.

Look better, feel better. One thing everyone's been taught since youth is to always feel good about yourself. Though you may not dwell too much on this idea, it's actually a life changing mentality that can differentiate an optimist and a pessimist. Thinking positively about yourself is the key to a happier life for anyone's situation before accepting anyone else except yourself for who you are. If you can't do that, then make yourself the person you want to be and accept that if you feel negatively about yourself, it'll be hard to see anyone else positively without choking on your own spite.

Negativity is an awful quality to have, but unfortunately it is more contagious than positivity. So if you walk around with a hunched back and a grumpy expression all day, it's highly likely you're dampening someone else's mourning. Even if that wasn't your intention, rather than being the party pooper, try being the life of the party. Make yourself a more confident and happier person by working on the most important part of your life. You're self functional fitness. Isn't that demanding of a dedication? All you need to do is honor fifteen to thirty minutes of your time. Focusing them on yourself may sound rude, but the truth is everyone gets conscious about their physique at some moment in their life.

Maybe it'd hit you in high school. Your coworkers unintentionally made broad shoulders part of the uniform, or your in-laws pointed it out a little louder than they should have. In any case, the idea isn't to feel bad about yourself, but to feel motivated to do something about it with little pushes. In the beginning, the results will start slipping into your jeans. Easier to show under your old sweaters and shirts and make your belts fall. Then by that time you'll be able to work harder for stronger results that will truly wow your audience, though the steps to get there aren't small, they are possible and not hard to walk.

Some great results from functional fitness are height and strength in your joints and limbs, greater resistance against physical impacts and a better posture. That's right. With all the work you're inputting to your joints and limbs, your posture will be heavily impacted. A straighter back, a courageous lift underneath your chin and strong shoulders. All kinds. From 15 minutes of functional fitness, every day is not something worth working for.

Functional Fitness & Other Exercises

In this chapter, we'll discuss functional fitness and other exercises. Functional fitness is commonly mistaken for any ordinary exercise and implemented into most typical workout chapters without anyone even realizing what it is. The fact is, there's a difference between functional fitness and other exercises, though the line between them may not be fully distinguishable at the moment. That'll all be cleared with the following comparisons between functional fitness and other types of exercises you may be familiar with. One Body-building Body-building focuses less on the daily routines and easing their exhaustion for you and more on the appearance you'll have in the end, no doubt about it.

The final judgment after Body-building is a great one, but it doesn't compliment all functional fitness has to offer. There are similarities between the two types of workouts. They both do help make for a better, stronger, healthier physical appearance. One exaggerates it more than the other. A fit, appealing body is what you'll get. But when it comes to similarities, that's all there is. Sometimes you may find some functional fitness moves in your bodybuilding workout, but you'll never find primary bodybuilding moves in a functional fitness routine. Functional fitness focuses less on grinding your muscles and more on your flexibility and higher standard strength in tasks you'll encounter when it comes to the daily routine.

Functional fitness is the helping hand holding you steady while you work through the day when you're a bodybuilder. Being the handy average Joe isn't what you're aiming for. Instead, it's more like you're aiming to be the extraordinary model people look up to and gaze appreciatively towards. Bodybuilders are built to appear tough, but the truth is that they're not that tough. When working on your muscles. The body builder way, the only thing you're doing is heightening the pulse and intensity of your muscles. Some core muscles in your limbs are completely skipped over and therefore not as strong as they could be.

So while a bodybuilder has the luck, they might not have the strength their muscles falsely portray. Bodybuilders are actually pretty delicate. They can't take hard impacts with swollen muscles and may have a harder time carrying themselves if they don't properly use their newfound power. When you're working out on a daily basis with the aim of greater performance ensures you'll achieve that goal. When you work to make the perfect vision, then by all means you'll get what you want. But then it's up to you to carry that proud physique to heavy weight training. This is no stranger to most people's vocabulary.

We've all seen the strong man in society lift the heaviest of weights with ease and blow our minds away. This is an extraordinary act indeed. But when will you ever do something that is out of the ordinary in your daily life? Functional fitness is quite similar to weightlifting and bodybuilding in various ways. You'll get the body and appearance you want, and most likely more than those of a normal functional fitness routine.

You'll also be able to lift amazingly heavy weights, which is great, right? I'm not. In every case in the gym, it might be a bragging right. Or when you're starting a conversation about your hard core hobbies. When it comes to working at home, though, lifting a box off the floor might strain your back painfully, even if it's a light box.

As mentioned earlier, functional fitness works on your daily life, making tasks you do each day easier and less of a hassle to perform steadily. Each chore becomes easier to do than the day before, when it was a bother. Functional fitness figuratively lightens the weights on your shoulders that were placed there. Weightlifters can easily lift weights off of their shoulders, but only when they are in the proper position with enough strength and utilizing the right equipment. Those who weightlift obviously know that there are protocols and conditions to be met when becoming weightlifters. How to prop yourself with the equipment, how to hold the bar of the dumbbell, and how to keep posture when holding the weights airborne.

These are all the things you prepare to do in weightlifting. An easier way to think of it is so when becoming a weightlifter, you are preparing for a foreseen event. That event is to gradually carry and handle heavier weights. When you're focusing on functional fitness, you're focusing more on preparing yourself for any possible event you'll encounter. So when it comes to practicality, functional fitness carries more weight, functional fitness targets, if not all, then most of the muscles you use on a daily basis by gradually strengthening them through a series of exercises, they become more efficient and perform to a higher degree.

When weightlifting, you only focus on strengthening those muscles, which will help you lift the heavy weights. This is fine as long as you're only planning on using those muscles for heavy lifting. The primary issue when it comes to weight lifting is the way you're doing it. You're either propped in a seated position or lying down in a steady pose that isn't going to harm the rest of your body. Doing this occasionally as weightlifters, would their muscles soon become accustomed to this formation? And this becomes the only formation in which they are working at peak performance when it comes to any formation, such as a. A very common example, heaving something from one surface to another, their formation back and muscles fail them, causing extreme pain. Three group training, when you're training by yourself in your own home, you have the luxury of comfort and solitude.

Anything you're doing suits your needs. All you have to do is make an environment that's fit for fitness and you're well on your way towards a healthy lifestyle. The making of your new person is done by your hand, which is pressure on no one else but yourself. What about when you work in a group? In a group you have an instructor which is a hefty pro since they know what they're doing in teaching. When you're working with a professional instructor, there's a greater environment of motivation to endure the workouts for a better appearance and healthier body. Those people around you could be friends or at least acquaintances that want to achieve the same goal as you making a friendly environment. The environment itself is one carefully designed to cater the needs of a workout. So you have the proper space, the proper colleagues and the proper instructor.

It sounds great so far. Now here's where the Hill drops. When you're working in a group, the catering isn't personal and generalized so that it fits a popular demand. Your demand may not be popular and you may find difficulty keeping up with the crowd. If you have a disability or any type of illness that prevents you from performing certain actions, you may as well not be part of the group when you're working by yourself. The workout can be adapted to suit all of your own needs and run to your own pace rather than the pace of others and an instructor who is already fit as a fiddle. So keep in mind all the time what it is you're looking for from your workouts to decisively decide what it is you need. And remember, functional fitness is a category of its own.

Common Mistakes With Functional Fitness

In this chapter, we'll talk about common mistakes with functional fitness, functional fitness is a great way to get yourself into shape so long as you're doing it right. If you're confused, then the easiest way to word it is you can work out wrong. There are many common mistakes most people make when they start working out by themselves or even when they're starting out in a gym. So before you start out on your own routine, take a look at some of the things that can go wrong before you make these very mistakes in everyday routine. One mistake people tend to make all too often is doing the same workout every single day. If you do this, you'll never get the ideal muscle tone and body that you want.

Yes. Over time, these workout chapters will get easier and you'll feel the strength in your limbs while doing this. But watch yourself crumble when you have to try a different workout. Your body is made up of many limbs, muscles, bones and joints. If you don't work on all these parts of your body equally, you'll end up with an imbalance in your strength and stamina which results in nothing good. Any good workout will have multiple actions that will target specific muscles in your body. When you combine the four main components of fitness discussed in later chapters, you get the right balance between everything your body needs. Unfortunately, this isn't as easy as piecing a puzzle together.

Instead, it's more like having to make smaller puzzles first in order to make a larger one. So when one workout focuses on cardio and perhaps muscle building, another workout you do through the week can focus more on HIIT and stretching. Keep switching up your exercises rather than doing the same one each day. Take it slow, only change your routine when you know you can handle new moves and challenges. If you constantly swap your daily exercise, you'll cover more ground quicker and spread the oncoming strength to all parts of your body. Only doing one type of exercise is going to tire you out and not properly help your body develop the way you'd have wanted it to. Love what you do, some people work out because they feel they have no other choice, no one can truly determine your own situation quite like you can. But this is the wrong mentality.

You should never approach your workout chapters with resentment. Always look at your workouts with optimism and confidence. If you want to work out, then do it for yourself, not for anyone else's satisfaction. If you feel that you're being pressured into working out, then the results are never going to satisfy you. Even if you do make it to your goal, you have to enjoy something in order to achieve anything. If you don't like cooking, then you'll never enjoy a meal. Even if you mastered the recipe. The victory is always sweeter when you've got sugar, not salt. Start working out when you feel good about working out.

Do workouts that make you feel confident, you have what it takes to make the change you need. If you don't like the criticism, comparisons or judgments of others, then don't go to the gym. You don't need to be in a crowd to get the motivation. You need to start lifting weights and running in the evenings. All your motivation should be positive, not negative. When you have positive motivation, it means you are being forward by the achievement you'll receive. When you have negative motivation, it means you are driven by the consequence of not acting. Don't be afraid of what people are going to say and do. If you don't work out, think about all the good responses you'll get from doing so.

Remember how happy you'll be when you finally reach where you want to be. Keep all of your thoughts positive and you'll not only feel good, but soon enough you'll look good as well. Dieting. Another one of the most common mistakes people make when they're starting out, they think they have to start dieting no matter what science and TV health programs try to tell you, dieting isn't the perfect solution for weight issues. Nowadays, people are coming to realize that diets actually limit you way too much. When you start dieting, you work with either elimination or restriction. This should never be the case. Eat as much as you can. Permit yourself to have a balance of everything edible out there.

Nothing should stop you from eating what you wish. Just have a balance with what you eat. Most of your normal diet should consist of healthy, hearty foods and whatever little snack your gluttony craves for can be satisfied once in a while. There is no issue with having a treat after some time. Keep control over how much junk food you have and keep that careful eye over your food to make sure the good always outweighs the bad. Working out doesn't make dieting compulsory. If anything, it means you have to keep yourself energized more often. You'll crave more food once you start working out and that craving is one you're going to want to satisfy. If not, you'll become grumpy, hungry, and your attitude towards working out won't be a very positive one.

Rolling with no goals. There's no race to be won. If there's no finish line. You always have to chart out your goals before you start working on a project. In this case, the project is yourself and you need to place some goals on what you want to do. Do you eventually want to have that hard core six pack? Are you aiming for a fitter, stronger? You lay out your goal and make it clear to yourself, otherwise you may as well be running headfirst into fog. Once you believe you have a goal set down, you're stepping stones to get there. You can't just hope you can make the jump from your side to the finish line, make the bridge and cross it one tile at a time. It's a timely process, but it'll grant you the guaranteed success you want.

It's better to work your way through at a decent pace rather than failing and having to restart the whole process. First, try to lose weight, aim for something that's fit and healthy, go for at least ten pounds less than what you are now. By the time you reach that goal, you'll have gotten accustomed to the fatigue and strain that follows a hefty workout chapter. You'll also have a stronger understanding of how much you can handle and where the limit can't be breached. Then try aiming for another goal. Seek to tone your muscles a little bit at first so you can understand how much time it takes you. Once you've gotten a clearer idea, you can start working hard on the final destination. All of this will take a decent amount of time, so don't give up. If the results don't show after weeks or maybe even a month, they'll come along soon. And once they do, it'll have been worth all of the time and effort.

Functional Fitness & Power

In this chapter, we'll talk about the first component of functional fitness power. When you first think of the word power, you may think of the word strength next. When it comes to working out, though, this isn't the case. Power and strength are two different aspects when it comes to exercise, each targeting and influencing different parts of the body. What is power? Power refers to your speed in doing something when you're performing an act at high speed and fluency such as jumping and running. This is referred to as your power. Power does have other meanings in other situations, such as the power or influence you have over someone or a certain situation.

But this does not apply to exercise. When you say that somebody is powerful in terms of their physique, you refer to the speed it takes someone to do something to clarify this point. Consider the following example. When you're capable of doing 50 pushups continuously, you're considered strong because of this capability. If you could do 50 pushups in two minutes, you'd be considered strong. But if the person next to you can do 50 pushups in half that time, they would be considered more powerful than you. The same applies even when you're competing in sports. If you're swimming, if you and another person can only do five laps in one go, you're both as strong as each other. But if the person swimming alongside you can do it in seven minutes while you do it in 10, they're more powerful than you. You can have the same level of strength as someone, but not the same level of power.

Having the same amount of strength as someone isn't that hard to achieve, as you may think, when it comes to having the same amount of power, though, it becomes very challenging to find someone on the exact same level as you. Don't get the wrong idea, though. Power and strength are both connected. Power is actually a combination of speed and the strength you have in order to do something without adequate strength, you won't have any power to exert. You'll also find that over a period of time, you'll lose your power faster than you lose your strength. This is because over time your body adjusts to wielding the strength it has. But as your body's original shape deteriorates over the years, your joints and muscles don't react as quickly as they would have done before.

Power is much harder to maintain than your level of power. The most common way to enhance your power would be by applying heavier weights to your workout so that you can perform your actions with greater resistance. To further understand why you need to maintain your level of power. Think of all the places where you need to be quicker and have more speed. Power in your daily life. Have you ever watched the public bus drive past when you need to catch it and break into a run? This is where your power would heavily influence whether or not you catch that bus. Most people have the strength to run across the street, but not everyone has the power to run across the street fast enough to catch the bus. If you do, then all is good for you. You'll reach work on time. But for those who don't.

Something has to change. Perhaps getting a car or you can develop greater power to enhance your strength and speed with all things you do. There's a certain amount of strength and ability required moving around. Items in your house require strength you may not use on a daily basis. Cleaning, for example, sweeping and dusting depend on a consistent movement of swaying your arm to and fro. You can have this strength to do so continuously, but do you have the power to do it quickly enough with power becomes more valuable time in your grasp. How so? Think of all the things you have to do in one day.

There are some things that will inevitably take time, like driving during traffic, waiting on the elevator and holding your spot in line during rush hour at the cafe. But during the day there are things you can control, such as climbing the stairs, walking or even getting ready in the morning. If you can better the actions you have control over every day, you can spare yourself more time and energy for those things beyond your control. With more time, you'll also have more stamina for the rest of your day. Some people are pooped after their daily morning routine, and if that's you, then there's no way you're getting through the day on an energized, positive principle. You shouldn't be crawling on all fours to get through your day.

You should be walking with stride each day, invigorated and prepared for the following days. This is why you need power throughout your day. You don't have to be a strong man to have power. Any ordinary person can enhance their power to become a better, more efficient version of themselves. Through progressive workouts. You can improve your performance. Think of power as the applications on a device to ease your understanding. Your phone would be your strength. With your phone, you're able to call people anywhere you go with applications, you're allowed to do more at faster speed to have access to social media and games. The more applications you have, the more you can do in less time. With only a phone, you have a base with applications you build up on that base to make it stronger.

Power moves a note to remember when it comes to most exercise moves, they've already combined all four components of functional fitness into the exercise. The following exercises are examples of those that you can use to gain benefit in all fields, including power, with these reasons further explained. One jump squats, jump squats are great for enhancing your core and leg power. This gives you the strength to withstand the resistance of squatting or simply bending down. With this move, you can bend your knees easier, knees being a primary area that wears out the fastest, you don't have to jump in this move. If it's your first time, you could simply squat to alleviate the strain of this motion to dumbbell curl. This move is by far the easiest to introduce to your workout.

Take one dumbbell in each hand and curl your arms at a steady pace. This helps you improve your general arm strength. With this, your arms won't succumb to heavy burdens when you pick up larger objects. The dumbbell curl can be made harder by holding your positions longer, introducing squats alongside the move, or by lifting the dumbbells over your head and then dropping them before curling your arms. Of course, all of these moves should be done after you're properly accustomed to regular dumbbell curves. Three ply lateral lunges. Rather than the usual lunge facing forward, take your lunges to the side, stand straight with your arms down, move your left leg outward to the left, stretch your left leg out so that it is straight, but your right leg is bent and go as far down as you comfortably can.

This will help your legs adapt to a sign of movement and strain from the upper body. This can help with extending your leg and bending down. When you feel comfortable with this move, introduce weights or resistance bands under your straightened leg. This will help the build up of power in your legs. For Burpee, this move is both as classic as it is functional. Your entire body's accustomed to general strain, from crouching to bending down to jumping all in one fluent move. Start by going down with your knees bent to your chest and then pump them out so you're in a planking position. After doing this, bring your legs back to your chest and jump upwards as soon as you land flat on your feet. Repeat this cycle to make this slightly more challenging. Bring your knees up to your chest while you're jumping. That way, your jumps have a stronger spring to them.

Functional Fitness & Strength

In this chapter, we'll talk about the second component of functional fitness strength next on the list of components is the mighty force of strength. Strength is what most people tend to pay attention to, though it isn't the only thing that makes you a stronger person as a whole. Strength is the foundation. You want to be sturdy and reliable in order for you to build over it. What is strength? Strength has been mentioned in the previous chapter quite a bit, but never properly defined. Strength when it comes to fitness is defined as exerting force against some kind of resistance. Everyone has their own level of strength, some greater and some lesser. In your daily life.

If you pay close attention to all you do, you'll come to realize that there are many times when you apply strength. You'll also notice that not all strength is the same. There are different types of strength that you apply every day, those being one maximum strength. This is the most amount of strength you can possibly exert in one go. Rolling your sleigh down the chapter, you'll want to have used your maximum strength to get the best push down for more fun. It's all you can do in the moment and if you have great strength levels, that's a lot of fun. Down the hillside to elastic strength, this one needs slightly more explanation.

Think of an elastic band and how fast it reacts when you let it go. It reacts similar to a whiplash for a fast and extremely hard impact. When you have elastic strength, that means you're capable of reacting to resistance with a fast or elastic contraction. Three Strength endurance. This is the ability to repeat an action over and over at the same consistency. Think of a baseball player mainly looking at the pitcher. Every time they throw the ball, they're expected to throw it at the same speed and force as the last time they did before. This is where you'll note their strength, endurance, all these types of strength have their own focused exercises that help enhance your durability in these fields. Without these strengths, there'd be a lot you wouldn't be able to do that can also be specialized in.

So if you only work on your strength and endurance, you may not have optimum elastic strength. When it comes to all strength training, you focus on the muscles connected directly to your bones. These are the muscles that work directly with your movements and therefore have a greater impact on how strong the outcome of your movement is. Strength training is often the first item on any workout list, since it's the foundation of all physical ability. When you have a sturdy enough base, you can move on to other focal exercises that center other objectives to be dealt with. If strength training isn't what you primarily targeted, then you may encounter issues with other workouts that turn out to be specialized in focusing on other functional aspects.

Strength in your daily life. You don't have to go to the gym to be strong. Strength applies to all aspects of our life. You can be emotionally strong, mentally strong, socially strong and more. In this case, you're concentrating on your physical strength. Physical strength is used in every move you make. When you walk, run, jump, heave and shove, you're using your strength to do so. When heaving large boxes, you'll be using your maximum strength when picking one up. After that, it's maintenance of your strength level to carry the box to where it needs to be. If you do this action over and over again, you'll be using your strength, endurance to withstand the constant strain created by the additional weights. If, for instance, the box slips from your hands while you're walking, you use your elastic strength to stabilize your grip.

As soon as your box starts slipping, your reaction, timing and elastic strength would work together to make sure you don't completely drop the box. All of your strengths work together every day to make sure you're always ready to take the load of the day. Another thing to note is that not all strength is trained with weights, but mainly resistance. Making the break between your exercises and repeating actions intensely are great ways to enhance your performance. Core workouts in complex chapters with greater variety all cover the muscles you need to bulk when working out strength. Workouts should never be intense when you're starting out, they should be easy, low level workouts with minimal variety. Your body needs to.

Accustomed to the new impact the workout is going to leave on you. You might have to take a break for the next one or two days if you're starting a new strength move. Strength exercise should always target your entire body since strength has to be your foundation for. All your physical activities, it's better if you get all the body parts pumped and ready for action in one go, most exercise moves that emphasize strength will recommend the use of weights. So when it comes to creating a heavy strength exercise, routine weights, resistance bands and yoga balls are your keys to finding the right way to truly test your limits. One single leg bridge. In this move, you'll be coordinating your leg and core for dual coverage. Lying face up, lift your leg until it's at 45 degrees into the air. Then lift your stomach a little to raise your leg higher.

This move should be done as a pump so that there's more burne with each repetition. This move helps coordinate the core with the legs, resisting strain and pressure. You can implement this move with a crunch or with leg weights to make it more intense to split squat. With this squat, you make it harder for yourself, creating more strain and resistance. For this move. You're not going to need weights, but a chair placing the chair behind you, place your foot on it so that one leg is bent and the other is straight. Then step forward and squat with the leg not on the chair. Do this with the other leg, swapping them to and fro until you feel the intense burn.

This means the workout is working and you're developing better leg strength. Three Glute Bridge. With this move, what you'll be doing is lying down on your back and lifting your glute only in a pump movement. This will strengthen your core as a whole for whenever you're going to bend or stretch your stomach, you can place weights in your hands while lifting your stomach, lifting the weights to increase both your arm and core strength for bent knee catchphrase. For this workout, you're going to need a box to step over, stand straight on your box, arms straight down and legs spread shoulder width apart. Have a weight in each hand while they hang, lift one of your legs up and bend slightly down on the one still on the box. Do this on each leg, one after the other for greater effect.

Functional Fitness & Range Of Motion

In this chapter, we'll talk about the third component of functional fitness range of motion next. Along the list of what contributes to your functional fitness workout is your range of motion. Your range of motion is defined as the measurement of movement around a specific body part. What is the range of motion? Think of how far you can stretch your leg over the stairs. You might be able to stretch your leg to the second step. You might make it to the third. If you're tall enough, stretch all the way to the fourth. But keep in mind, you're using your range of motion as you're doing. This range of motion can be associated with your flexibility, but they aren't entirely the same thing. Flexibility is the abstract movements your body can perform. Range of motion is quite literally the range of how far you can go.

So when you work on your flexibility, you're also working on extending your range of motion. Your range of motion is what allows you to extend your reach and keep your limbs alive, ready and always moving. Your range of motion relates to how well you can move around, how far your reach can go. Being strong is great, but if you can't reach the top shelf without stretching a muscle, then you're missing out on a few vital exercises. Range of motion mainly comes from stretches. You should occasionally stretch your limbs in all directions where you can comfortably go. This way, you keep a hold of your range of motion.

Range of motion is as easy to lose as your power is. Once you've lost the flow or routine of strengthening, it's really hard to get it back. Range of motion may not seem that important on its own, but combined with the other components of functional fitness, it really makes the difference between one person and another. You may have immense power and strength, but without a decisive range of motion, you'll never be the best runner. Since your legs aren't accustomed to taking such large steps with power and strength, you can run consistently at a fast pace, which is good to make yourself better. You can improve the length of your stride by stretching your legs during exercises. Never think of the components of functional fitness on their own because on their own they aren't worth much.

When they work together, they create a strong, sturdy base that you can rely on every single day. Range of motion in your daily life. Range of motion applies to everything you do, though you may not notice it in your daily actions. When you stretch to reach something overhead, when you take a longer stride to step over a puddle, when you kneel down to find something hidden under your bed. They're all examples of range of motion in your life. When you work on your range of motion, you not only work on extending your reach, but also are making it easier for you to reach that far. Think of what happens. The further you reach, it'll be easier to run, jump and walk at a faster pace. You can stretch overhead and blow yourself effortlessly.

Actions in general become much easier when you work out. You do actions in a more exaggerated manner than what they really are in real life. This technique ensures that anything you do in your daily routine remains something easily doable rather than a brother that'll hurt your back after doing it. Range of motion isn't something you work on on its own. It's interpreted with everything you do in real life. And in your workout chapter, though, you'll find workouts that convey they are primarily a range of motion workouts. They'll actually have a secondary focal point that additionally trains your range of motion.

The best part about training a range of motion is that it can be as easy as stretching in the morning after you wake up, roll over to the side of the bed and stretch your arms over your head, rattle your legs a little bit and arch your back. All of these can help day by day to make you reach a little better than it was yesterday. Have a yoga chapter, go out for a run. Doing the smallest of things can help your range of motion. The more you do it, the greater its development. So as long as you endlessly keep at it every day for even fifteen minutes, you'll feel and see the difference the next time you reach for the top shelf.

Range of motion moves, these actions are better done in between at the beginning and in the end of your workout, all of these moves are done better when you hold them for a minimum 20 seconds, each one lunges with a spinal twist. It's the usual lunge with a new twist for you to try out. Once you're in the lunge stance, place one hand down on the floor and the other in the air, twisting your core so that you're facing upwards, turning between your arms, taking your movements slowly. This helps your core leg and arm stretch. All is done in one move and the longer you hold it, the stronger the burn and the easier it'll be the next time you do it. Two butterflies stretch rather than stretching your limbs outwards.

Bring them all inwards so that you're comfortable in closed positions. Sit down and bring your feet together, making them touch each other's souls. Place your right hand on your left shin and your left hand on your right shin. Keep this pose for as long as you can. Standard 20 seconds to have the best effect. Three seated shoulders squeeze in this move, you're sitting on the floor quite like how you did in the butterfly stretch, only this time you take your arms to your back and clasp them together immediately. You should feel your shoulder bones constraining in the pose.

Functional Fitness, Balance & Endurance

In this chapter, we'll talk about the fourth component of functional fitness, balance and endurance. Finally, to complete the set of four, there's the last and final component, balance and endurance. These two work together in all ways and help enhance everything you can do, including the other components mentioned earlier. What is balance and endurance? Balance and endurance? Both have separate definitions. Balance is defined as your capability to control, handle and manage your body's movement. There are two types of balance to consider, those being your static balance and your dynamic balance. Static balance refers to the balance you must acquire while you're stagnant completely.

Still, this type of balance is easier to learn to control over your dynamic balance, which is your level of balance when you're mobile. In addition to balance would be coordination, which is a very important theory in fitness coordination is the capability to do two or more things at once. Move your body in two or more different ways with fluency and efficiency. Balance and coordination go hand in hand and held in your other hand would be endurance. Endurance, which can also be referred to as stamina, is the ability of your muscles and body to remain active during a lengthy period of time. Together, balance and endurance help create a set time limit of how long you can do something with good balance and standard endurance. You'll be active for a long amount of time. This leads to the final summary of all the components of functional fitness.

With the proper amount of strength, you have a solid base to become a fit person. Your strength is going to help you withstand all the restraint you'll experience while you're working out. Power is the speed that you can apply to your workouts to handle them quicker and with more force. Power helps build up your strength so that there's more to exert helping you reach the extra mile. The other way you're going to reach the extra mile is by using your range of motion, which is going to help you reach further in a shorter amount of time. Don't get power and range of motion confused. Power will take you faster. Range of motion will take you further. Together, they create a useful duo. Finally, there's your balance and endurance there.

The components that give you a time limit on how long you can last at peak performance, there's a limit to everything and eventually you'll wear down. Your balance will falter and your breath harsher and raspier put them all together and you have all the pieces to create the perfect, complete puzzle to understanding your maximized personal health. Balance and endurance in your daily life balance and endurance keep you running through the day in the most minimal way they go together as well as rhymes, do harmoniously ensuring that you have the equity and stamina to progress through the events occurring all day, every day. As the saying goes, everything works when there's a balance.

The simplest and most relatable example would have to be when going up the stairs while going up the stairs. Each moment you lift your foot is a split second of momentary balance. In this case, you'll also require the stamina to keep going up flights of stairs with the right amount of stamina. You can make it up the entire staircase, but without it you'll be wheezing after the third flight. Balance and endurance are actually two things you can't notice quite easily. These two attributes keep improving on a daily basis and contracting at the same time. The more you do in one day, the better you'll be tomorrow. The less you do today, the less you'll be able to do tomorrow.

If you consistently improve your balance and endurance, you'll consistently get better results. But balance, coordination and endurance aren't aspects you can simply stop working on. As soon as you find yourself on a suitable level of endurance, you keep at it, maintain your level and never fall from it. As you get older, it'll be harder to keep one level. So it's better to maintain rather than trying to climb any higher just as well. If you stop working on them, your balance and endurance are going to fall by the day. Cleaning, cooking, walking, talking. These are all things that take up your endurance, running, heaving. Any sort of movement with any part of your body all requires some balancing effort.

Without proper care, walking will become a chore and you'll become lethargic without the right level of stamina, balance and endurance moves. When it comes to these kinds of workouts, you're easily staring down some balance moves of all shapes and sizes. You can even have a full yoga chapter once or twice a week to cover this type of workout. One one leg stand. In this workout, you'll be standing with one leg airborne in the other, one rooted to the floor. Try holding this pose for as long as you can. At first you might want to hold on to a wall or chair so you can better adjust to the pose. If your balance is generally not good, then start with your arms stretched outwards for greater balance. If you have better balance, then complicate this easy step by pumping your elevated leg. This way you can better both your balance and your power with one move.

To plunge in this version of a lunge, every time you bend down over one leg, you're going to jump and swap to the other leg. In this manner, you're going to help enhance your endurance with each swap, imitating the actions you do when running Pleyel. Lunge is more intense than a normal lunge. So please don't try it unless you're comfortable and more than capable of doing a regular lunge. First three straight leg catchphrases. Would this move? Your balance will be intensely tested, standing on a step or box with your heels hanging over the edge. Lift one leg behind yourself. Push your foot up so that you're on your toes. Hold for a few seconds and then come back down. Swap your legs after a few bumps on each foot. This is going to hurt when you do it, but you'll surely have better balance after this.

Recap

There's no perfect way to work out. Everyone has different needs and requirements, so there are different goals and ambitions that are always being followed. Not everyone wants to be a bodybuilder, and some people would rather know how to lift weights in the gym.

More than anything, what you want is what should be most important to you. Your goals should be reached if you want them to be. So never falter your beliefs in yourself and take it the slow and simple way, the functional fitness way.

With all the effort you put into yourself, the right amount of balance in everything you do and the courage to step up no matter what happens, you'll surely get what you need in the end to run. You have to know how to walk to stop. You have to have started first to function. You have to better prepare your own health, your own functional fitness.

Kettlebell

Kettle Bells is one of the exercises that most people regard as cool and interesting, if you have not seen a kettlebell before, you may be curious what it looks like. Well, it's pretty straightforward. It is a black cannonball with a handle that is cast of iron. Well, there are so many other workout tools that you can employ to achieve your health goals. One thing that you have to appreciate is that the kettlebell training has a unique factor and that is a good enough reason to incorporate it into your workout routine. Part of what makes kettlebell exercises, Mystikal, lies in its origin. They debuted in Russia in the 18th century.

During this time, the kettlebell was used as counterweights when measuring things like cereals and other dry products. Soon enough, the farmers started challenging each other to lift the heaviest kettlebells, and eventually they found their way into the hands of strong circus men. After the Second World War, the Soviet Red Army took up the kettle in training their soldiers and later in the 1970s, lifting kettlebells was declared an official sport. Well, kettle bells have been around in the U.S. for over a century, they have enjoyed its fair share of resurgence and eventually found their way into the gym and fitness stores. It comprises a bell, a handle and Hornes.

The bell in this case refers to the round cannonball shaped weight, and the handle is what connects the kettlebell by simply sloping downwards on the end, hence referred to as the horns. It is the design that makes the kettlebell quite a unique tool, you may be thinking, what is the difference between kettlebells and dumbbells? Well, one thing you have to take note of is that unlike the dumbbells in which the handle connects to weights that are evenly distributed and lies at the center of them, the kettlebell center of gravity is usually offset from its handle. This is mainly because it rests several inches away from the center.

It is also important to note that with a kettlebell, it is quite easy to grasp it by the handle bell, end or horns, it is the mainstay to grip the kettlebell by its handle. However, when it comes to certain exercises like squats, it is much easier to grasp them by the horns to achieve a greater grip on certain poses like rowing. It may be better to hold the kettlebell by the bell itself. This is because it will help force the hand to squeeze harder to prevent slipping.

How to Properly Choose A Kettlebell

In this chapter, we'll talk about how to choose a kettlebell. According to a study conducted at the University of Wisconsin, La Crosse, there are so many ways in which you can choose a kettlebell, mostly the kettlebell, vary and designs. There are those that are coated with rubber to protect the floors from the resulting impact, other designs are designed specifically for competitions. Such cattle bells have a straight handle and are uniform in shape and size, irrespective of the weight. Over the years, some manufacturers have designed kettlebells with a concave face for ergonomic factors. Others, like the new fangled kettlebells, worked the same way as dumbbells, which means that they can be loaded with plates to offer multiple weight changes with just a single implement.

For instance, kettlebell swings and getups are said to get the heart rate up and burn more fat in the same manner a cardio machine does, but can do more in reinforcing good mechanics. Therefore, if you plan on buying a kettlebell in person, it is important that you do the test before making up your mind, start by holding up your hand and touch your thumb to the tip of your pinky. Take note of the channel this forms on your palm, this is the point at which the kettlebell handle is supposed to rest most of the time, that is from the outside knuckle of your index finger down to the opposite side of your wrist in a diagonal orientation. Follow this by picking up the weight and then holding the handle in the middle so that it fills the channel, ensuring that the bell rests on the back of your forearm and that the wrist at this point is straight.

It's important that it does not impinge on the bony profile of your wrist. If at some point you pick up the kettlebell and it rubs against the bone protruding on the lateral side of your wrist, then this means that the weight displacement from the handle is not ideal. In other words, there is a high risk of you getting injured. The best safety tip at this point is to avoid choosing a kettlebell that has a thick handle, you will realize that on its handles have a diameter that is a little over an inch. This is enough when it comes to working your grip, but not as demanding to hold and so does not create unnecessary fatigue.

When performing an exercise like a swing, there is a possibility that you will be making so many reps in a single workout. The key here is to ensure that your grip does not burn out. This is mainly because it is counterproductive from a technical standpoint, when the grip is overworked, there is a chance that you will see a whole slew of mechanical problems that will occur. As for how much weight you should begin with, men can do 16 kilos, while women can do eight kilos.

Benefits of Kettlebell Training

In this chapter, we'll talk about the benefits of kettlebell training. There are so many benefits that you get to enjoy by performing kettlebell workouts. One thing that is important to note is that kettlebell training offers a unique combination of benefits from strength exercises when using the kettle bells and those from cardio. As mentioned earlier, a kettlebell workout is more unconventional and quite resembles a cannonball with a handle attached to it. You can use it to build your strength, agility, boost balance and endurance while at the same time promoting weight loss. Kettlebell exercises often feature a wide range of lifts and swings. The good thing is that the training tool is quite flexible and can be used for a broad range of intense training exercises.

Therefore, if you need a hybrid system for both strength and cardio, the kettle bells are your best option at creating workouts that are not only effective but also time efficient. So if you are still weighing whether or not to ditch those unconventional dumbbells for something that will be worth your while, here are some of the benefits that you do not want to miss when you choose kettlebell training. One, to achieve better form, one of the main things that distinguish a kettlebell from a dumbbell usually lies in the offset nature of the load.

This is mainly because the center of gravity of a kettlebell is about six to eight inches away from your grip when you are holding the handle. And this is what makes it quite difficult to control. Because of this, every exercise that you perform, ranging from conventional strength movements to more unique kettlebell exercises such as swings, you are going to need a strict form and an increased activation of the muscles that you could get from using a dumbbell. Let us consider an overhead press in this case, one of the funniest things when using a dumbbell is the fact that so many people are as happy to press at the point where their elbows are bent at a right angle.

However, with kettlebells, the first instinct is to press up to lockout. This is mainly because the offset load serves as a counterweight that plays a critical role in pulling the shoulders back. In other words, the kettlebell plays a significant role in encouraging you to perform each exercise optimally and perfectly. However, if you cannot, for instance, you end up arching your back or twisting to one side when trying to complete the lift, then you most certainly know that your form is broken. When you squat with a kettlebell held in front of your body, this causes you to sit back and this improves the mechanics of your squat pattern tremendously. This, in effect, paves the way for you to progress to more advanced exercises seamlessly when the time comes.

Two improves your core strength when you press the kettlebell overhead, you are simply causing your ribs and back to flare. This means that you have to lock your car as much as you can to prevent it from happening. When you are in a swing, it is critical that you brace your car to prevent your lower back from dangerously rounding at the bottom of the movement's. Therefore, for each exercise you perform, the good thing is that you can count on your core firing harder with the aim of stabilizing your body and ensuring that your safety comes first.

Three boost athleticism, if you are an athlete, one of the major benefits of incorporating KETTLEBELL in your workout routine is the fact that you gain a greater grip strength. This is mainly because the kettlebell handle, together with the displaced load, needs your hands, fingers and forearms to work harder and control it than when using a dumbbell. While so many manufacturers prefer thick handles, one thing that you have to understand is that when you use a narrower handle, you are making it quite easy to perform complex movements. This increases your training options.

Because grip strength is much more significant than in most sports, as well as gaining overall strength, kettlebells have the opportunity of boosting your cardiovascular endurance. Kettlebell exercises often incorporate the whole body and such workouts as the press snatch and clean involve lifting weights right from the floor to over the head. This ensures that the muscles across the body are worked well and these motions create a huge demand on the heart. As a result, so many athletes employ the use of kettlebells as a strong pillar of their workout programs for easy portability, just like exercise bans and suspension trainers, kettlebells are quite portable and it's easy to bring them with you on travel. This is because they will not roll around in your car as dumbbells do.

They will not look odd at all when you bring them to the beach with you. Additionally, unlike the dumbbell, you only need one kettlebell for you to have a great workout. This is because with just a single kettlebell, you can engage in a large number of exercises, unlike the dumbbell, that you mostly need at least a few selections of them to do your regular workouts.

If you intend on working the entire body, you can choose to bring with you to kettlebells. The truth is, if you have a single kettlebell at the corner of your room or the back of your car, you pretty much have a gym. Five lower body fats. So many people desire to shut off a few pounds and hence weight loss is one of their major fitness goals.

The good thing with kettlebell training is that you can achieve this and more. The main reason for this is the fact that kettlebell training integrates a large number of high intensity workouts that allows the body to burn as much fat as possible. While so many weight loss programs take too much time and effort to achieve the desired body weight and physique and end up becoming boring over time, kettlebell training is quite the opposite. This is mainly because it serves as an exciting alternative to your average routine workouts, because they keep you focused and boost the rate of your metabolism.

It is highly recommended that if you intend to lose weight using kettlebell training, you integrate high repetition compound movement exercises in every chapter. Some of these exercises may include reverse lunges, kettlebell swings and shoulder presses. The most important thing is to ensure that you do not have rest times in between. Six improves posture. One of the things with the human body is that as age progresses, our posture is also affected. However, the good thing is that you can make sure that you control the effects of aging by incorporating kettlebell training into your workout routine.

This is because, according to research, there is evidence that shows kettlebell exercises can improve posture and counter the effects of modern day lifestyles. Well, working out, it is very common for postural muscles to be neglected, but with kettlebell training, you can dramatically improve the results and boost the posture. Do you know why this is important? Well, an improved posture helps you look leaner and boost your self-esteem and confidence. Seven inexpensive. The other good thing with kettlebells is the fact that they are cost effective. When you buy the right kettlebell, you can be sure that they will last a lifetime and you will not need to incur another cost of replacing them frequently.

For most beginners, getting a single kettlebell that is made from solid metal can last for so many years. Moreover, kettlebell training does not need you to be in specialized footwear like other workouts. And this ensures that you save money that you would have otherwise spent on purchasing an expensive pair of workout shoes. Eight gaining strength without bulk. Did you know that most women who work out possess a common desire to build their strength without necessarily having a bulky appearance of a male bodybuilder? Well, with kettlebell training, the main aim is not to increase the muscle mass, but to boost strength without having that bulky appearance.

This is mainly because when you integrate the kettlebell exercises to your training program, you are essentially incorporating full body functional movements. These movements play a central role in simultaneously targeting many muscle groups across the body. If you have any special needs, it is advisable that you talk to your trainer about them so that they can design workout routines that satisfactorily meet these requirements. Nine are comfortable to use, unlike dumbbells that have a high chance of straining your arms and other workouts that put you at risk of injuries, kettlebells are very comfortable to use.

This is mainly because they do not pull the muscles across the body too hard. Their weights rest comfortably in your forearms without weighing them down and causing fatigue. This explains why women prefer using kettlebells than other weight lifting exercises available. Ten quick workouts, most of us do not have enough time to sign up and hit the gym. However, this does not mean that there are no workout exercises that will keep your body in great shape.

Kettlebell exercises are perfect for you, and you can do them at the comfort of your home office or any other place that you are comfortable with. Kettlebell targets so many muscles in the body, and this means that you do not have to spend so much time on other workouts that only target one body part at a time. This is exactly what makes kettlebell training a brilliant solution for people who have busy schedules like Mom. Best of all, you can perform these workout exercises with minimal supervision.

Common Kettlebell Mistakes

In this chapter, we'll learn about the common kettlebell mistakes. So far, we have already discussed how kettlebell training is effective in building strength and power. It is also clear that there is a wide range of kettlebell training tools available in the market, each playing a significant fitness goal. For instance, the kettlebell swing plays an important role in boosting the body's endurance while also strengthening the posterior chain. However, one thing that you have to bear in mind is that with kettlebell training exercises, it is not always fun and games if you are a beginner.

It is critical that you pay attention to what you are doing and how you are doing it to minimize the occurrence of injuries. If you are just starting to ensure that you get the guidance that you need from an expert fitness coach to help you learn how to use the kettlebell equipment the right way. Here are some of the common mistakes that you should look out for when using the kettlebell. Mistake one, opting for a heavier weight when starting it is very easy for one to get caught up with so much excitement and the temptation to push yourself too hard.

Yes, the challenge is good, but you have to do it gradually so that the body is not in shock. In other words, rather than jumping all in to start off with heavier weights than you can handle, it is important that you start with what you can handle and progress slowly when you add more weight than you can handle. You will only restrict in an improper form and increase the risk of having an injury. Whenever you are training, always ensure that your safety comes first, the best way to do this is ensuring that you select the right kettlebell weight of kettlebell.

Consult with a professional when you decide to choose the weights, to start training with, ensure that you are not mixing up the measurements and weights by learning the difference between meters and centimeters and pounds and kilograms. Mistake to generating force by using the upper part of the body. As mentioned earlier, the kettlebell exercises often utilize movements of the whole body. This is what makes the training chapters twice as effective. Unfortunately, there are so many people at the beginner level who try hard to muscle up their way through these workouts, it is important that you realize how this might place unnecessary strain on your upper body and try not to do it.

Mistake three, swinging the kettlebell too fast. One important thing you have to understand is that when you swing the kettlebell too fast, you risk losing control and pulling your muscles, something that could result in serious injuries. While it is often exciting to swing the kettlebell with so much force after a very long day. There is a chance that this might do more harm than good to your form. Mistake for focusing on quantity. As a beginner, there is a high chance that you will be tempted to go overboard and push yourself too hard if your trainer recommends that you start with 10 reps. Going higher than this isn't a good idea.

Trust me, finishing 20 reps with bad form is even worse than never picking up a kettlebell simply because you are employing the wrong kind of technique. It is essential that you perform each kettlebell exercise as it is required so that you avoid the adverse effects that might cause injury, adhere to guidelines before you can even attempt to perform any exercise at all. Mistake five, putting on the wrong running shoes, like I mentioned earlier, the good thing is that you do not have to wear a special kind of shoe to do this exercise. However, this does not mean that you can wear a shoe that places you at a risk of injury.

While it is tempting to wear a shoe with a very thick skull, you have to understand that this might hinder your movements while working out when performing the kettlebell exercises. It is advisable that you wear a shoe that allows you to naturally move your ankles, lower leg, ligaments and foot. Thick running shoes do not only cushion the heels, but also tend to raise the foot off the ground, causing your grip on the floor to be destabilized.

Common Mistakes During Kettlebell Exercises

In this chapter, we'll talk about remedies to common mistakes during kettlebell exercises. Remedy one before you get your hands on any kettlebell. It is critical that you practice basic movements first. The best way to do this is by starting with a few mobility exercises just to warm the joints up. You can also start with lightweight objects like water bottles to practice kettlebell swings, especially if you are a beginner. This ensures that you learn mobility without having to put yourself at risk of injury. Remedy, too, for you to effectively and efficiently practice using the force derived from the whole body, it is critical that you consider practicing the kettlebell swings first.

This will go a long way in helping you experience power being transferred from the lower parts of your body to the upper parts. Just bear in mind that your back needs to be kept flat and your glutes squeezed, sooner or later you will be proficient performing kettlebell workout exercises with so much zeal. Remedy three, the next time you will be practicing the kettlebell swing, one of the things that you should pay attention to is doing it at a slower and controlled pace. This is very critical in stabilizing and strengthening the larger groups of muscles while lowering the risk of injuries. It is therefore very important for you to take control of the bell while moving it downwards, just as it is when moving upwards.

Just like any other exercise, kettlebell swings require you to control its movement when you bring it around the head and ensure that the shoulders are stable. Remedy for a beginner, it is advisable to start by simply setting yourself a small target, focus your attention on completing at least 10 reps before you can move higher than this. Once you can handle it, you can now add a small number of reps to your workout chapters bit by bit. It is better if you talk to your trainer about the problems you might be facing. Well, it's a good option to work out at home. It is important that you seek expert guidance, especially if you have never used the kettlebell before.

Remedy five, try as much as you can to do your kettlebell workouts while wearing flat shoes with a better grip of the floor. You could also choose to do the exercises in bare feet. When you get rid of shoes, you stand a chance of strengthening your feet, muscles and ligaments so that you have the freedom to move around seamlessly. Alternatively, you can choose to wear Converse, which has been proven to strengthen both the feet and the ankles.

Ways To Use Kettlebells

In this chapter, we'll discover ways to use kettlebells. There are three major ways in which you can use kettlebells when working out, these include warm ups. If you are just finding out that health and fitness is something that you should be focusing on and want to get back in shape, kettlebells are the best tool to avoid imbalances and injuries. This is mainly because they will warm up your body by simply restoring healthy movement patterns in your body. However, if you are not ready to start integrating cattle bells in your workout program, at least start using them little by little to enhance your mobility. This will help you get in position so that you can perform regular weight lifts safely. This means that when you begin to go for heavy loads, your body can handle it and you can maintain the technique.

Even though the kettle bells are much lighter than you think or what you are used to, they offer you adequate feedback to challenge yourself and light up your nervous system. This means that the communication between the body and the brain is enhanced and this boosts a more responsive system to what you are asking it to do. The trick is for you to try your best to do the goblet squats before you can proceed to back squats by simply holding the lower position for a couple seconds before opening up the hips. You can also try doing the light one arm overhead presses before progressing to military presses so that your shoulders stay warm. Alternatively, you can choose to use the chest loaded swings to make your hips ready for kettlebell deadlifts.

Doing full body workouts, all that you need for a great workout is to ensure that you are working all the major and minor muscles of your body. With kettlebells, you can achieve this using squats, hinge pull and push techniques, once you cover these movement patterns, you are good to go. Set a circuit when it comes to swings and getups, you are sure to get your heart rate up to the same rate you would in a cardio machine. The most important thing with the kettlebell is that you can do more to reinforce good mechanics. The other bright side is that while you exercise, you are challenging yourself to be better while having so much fun. The trick is for you to try as much as you can to build a circuit with kettlebells before you can progress to heavy weight training chapters.

Kettlebell Workouts For Beginners

In this chapter, we'll talk about kettlebell workouts for beginners. If you ask any trainer, they will tell you that kettlebells are here to stay because they have outstanding outcomes, it is the one workout technique that can work multiple joints all at the same time. It is the one technique that you can use to achieve so many results simultaneously. It is not only great for the heart and the core, but also offers the ability to stabilize the body. To warm up the body with this exercise begin by standing with your feet hip width apart, hold the kettlebell to your chest and then using your right hand, hold the corner of the kettlebell handle and lower down into a squat position.

Once you are in the squat position, begin to thread the bell in between your legs so that you reach behind and use your left hand to grip the corner of the handle. Now that the kettlebell is in your left hand, behind your left leg, start moving it along the outer parts of your left thigh, then start threading it back to the middle of your legs. But this time ensure that you grab it with your right hand and hold it behind your right leg. Again, start moving it around the right leg and then bring it to the front of your right hand as a beginner, you can start with at least five reps and then work your way up to 10 gradually once the body can handle it. One kettlebell swing, this is one of the most popular workout exercises that you should incorporate into your daily fitness routine to get the perfect kettlebell swing.

Start by standing over the kettlebell with your feet hip width apart and your chest up. Hold your shoulders back and then move down with the kettlebell lined between your feet. It is important that you invest in a kettlebell that permits you to swing using one of the perfect techniques without having to challenge yourself if you are a beginner. It is critical that you start with a lightweight kettlebell or use one that is way lighter than what you are used to. Now swat down while ensuring that you grip the kettlebell with your palms so that your thumb loosely grips around the handle and stands tall while gripping onto the kettlebell.

It is critical that you keep your arms long and loose enough to engage the core and cause the shoulder blades to retract. At this point, it is important that you start shifting the body weight toward your heels while keeping the knees softened, then slowly lower the rear end towards the wall behind you and then start swinging the kettlebell. Start driving your heels so that your quads are engaged while still swinging the kettlebell. It is critical that as you swing the kettlebell, it reaches your chest and the arms remain extended. As the bell begins to come down, words allow the wait to work the magic while you get ready for the next wrap, shift away toward your heels so that the glutes and the hamstrings are loaded and then the weight will move behind your legs.

While the bells transition from the back to the front, keep engaging your heels and your hips to maximize the benefits, repeat the whole process at least 10 times, and once you can handle it, you can gradually increase the reps. Two Turkish get up, this is one of the most commonly known full body workouts that integrates fundamental movement patterns that are important in conditioning, the stabilizer muscles and the core throughout the process. It is termed the best stabilizing exercise and has been used for so many decades in ancient Greece. It is believed that the Greek would not train a boy until they can get off the floor while holding the weights above their heads, this exercise entails seven stages.

Stage one starts by forming a fetal position while ensuring that you are holding the kettlebell, then roll onto your back and then hold the bell such that your arm is straightened out, fix your gaze on the kettlebell and ensure that your eyes are not taken off it. Stage to start bending your leg so that they are in the same direction as the kettlebell at the same time place your opposite arm such that it is at 45 degrees, stage three, once you are sighted along the line of your arm, crushed the handle to your elbow and then follow up with the hand start to position the kettlebell arm in its rightful socket. Stage four now starts pushing from the heel of your bent leg and then pushes your hips up so that they are fully extended, ensuring that there is a straight line running from the bottom hand to the bell.

Stage five, sweep the straight leg through and then back so that you are in a half kneeling position. Stage six, lift the hands off the floor and then begin to extend the body so that it is straight, take your eyes off the ball and focus on what lies ahead of you. Stage seven, drive slowly from your heel and stand straight up on your feet, once you achieve stability, you can reverse the movements and start from the beginning to the end for the number of replicates that is desired. Three Kettlebell Windmill, this is an exercise that is designed mainly for strengthening the core, it also plays a central role in decreasing the waistline.

Start by positioning the kettlebell at the front of your lead foot. Use your opposite arm to press overhead, clean the bell to your shoulder by simply extending through your hips and the legs such that the kettlebell moves in the direction of your shoulders. Start rotating the rest in such a way that the palms face forward and then press the kettlebell overhead by simply extending the elbows straight. In this position, ensure that you keep the kettlebell locked out so that you can push your glutes in the same direction as the locked bell, extend your feet to achieve a 45 degree angle from the arm while maintaining the kettlebell locked out while you bend the hips, begin to slowly lean forward until you reach the ground with your free hands.

While doing this, it is important that you keep your eyes gazing on the kettlebell throughout as you hold it over your head, take a 30 second pause once you reach the floor before you can get back to your starting position. For single leg deadlift, this exercise is important in helping you learn how to stabilize when in motion, it is critical that you practice this movement so that when you will be holding a kettlebell, you can swing it at high speed without tripping. It is a comprehensive exercise that plays a critical role in singling out your legs during the deadlift process. One thing that you have to bear in mind when engaging in this exercise is that it requires balance. It is also essential that you pay attention to your glutes, hamstrings and your lower back. Indeed, it is a great exercise that will help you achieve toned lean legs while strengthening your posterior chain.

The first thing that you have to do is position your feet together while you place the kettle bells on your toes, then pick it up while you use one leg and raise the other behind you. Maintain a straight back as you place the bell back to the floor and repeat the whole process for about five to 10 reps. One of the safety tips that should help you as you engage in this workout is to hold on to the kettlebell handle so tight while maintaining a tight core. As you do this, you should be able to feel the tension on both your hamstrings and your glutes.

Five kettlebell goblets, squat, the first thing that you do here is to hold accountable by the horns and then drive your shoulder blades towards each other and downwards towards the chest that the chest opens, then tuck your elbows in so that your forearms are in a vertical orientation. Stand with both your feet wider than hip width apart, ensure that the feet are slightly turned out and then take in deep breaths into your belly, start twisting your feet into the ground and take a squatting position while keeping your torso upright, go as low as possible without allowing your tailbone to tuck under your butt.

Six one arm overhead presses start by standing tall while holding the kettlebell in one hand at the level of your shoulder, standing firmly with your feet rooted into the ground as though you were getting ready to resist a push. Taking deep breaths into your belly and ensuring that you brace your glutes and abs. Now, pull your ribs down so that your spine looks elongated and your chest is out and the tailbone is slightly tilted. Start pressing the weight overhead, it is important that you ensure your chin is pulled back so that the weight clears it easily. Now, lower the kettlebell by pulling it back into position as though you were performing a pull up.

It is important that you do not get fixated on getting the overhead lockout immediately, you have to understand that achieving the right angle elbow bend is not easy for most people. Therefore, if you see, you need to answer back so that your ribs can flare, do it. This will help you lock out the arms overhead so that the shoulders train effectively. In most cases, you might find it necessary to regress the movements towards the ground by simply lying down on the floor with your triceps against it, then pressing upwards from there as though you were doing a bench press, only this time with a shortened range of motion.

Seven kettlebell deadlifts start this exercise by placing the kettle bells on the floor in between your feet. Now stand with your feet hip width apart slightly, bend the knees so that you can push your butt back. Ensure that your feet are rooted to the ground while you try to lower your torso until your arms can grip onto the kettlebell handle. With your chest out, keep your back as naturally arched as possible. It is important that you let your eyes gaze in front of you, but slightly lower, then grasp the kettlebell using both your hands and then take a deep breath into your belly. Now drive through your heels and lift the bells while you extend your hips to lockout.

Eight kettlebells, one arm row. Start by placing the kettlebell down on the floor and then place your right foot in front as you take a staggered stance, plant your right foot outside your weight. Ensure that you plant the ball of your left foot into the ground and fold it at the hips as you bring yourself into a sitting position in such a way that your butt and torso are at a 45 degree angle to the ground, then rest your elbow on your right thigh for support. Then reach out for the kettlebell with the help of your left hand. Inhale slowly into your belly as you draw your shoulders back and towards each other, brace your core as you throw the weight towards your hips, squeeze your shoulder blades together at the top and repeat the whole process for about eight to 10 reps.

Nine kettlebell goblets, half get up, just like the kettlebell swing worked out, so many people who use kettlebell prefer to skip ahead to moves that are more advanced than they can handle. Instead of jumping right in with a Turkish getup, which is quite complex, it is important that you understand that as a beginner, starting with a half get up still offers you an incredible core workout, just like any other flexibility workout. To do this, start by lying down on your back while holding the kettlebell by the horns, inhaling it softly into the belly while you brace your abs.

Now, start performing sit ups as you tuck your right foot towards your bed and then chapter your left foot behind you in such a way that you form something like a shin box while on the floor, ensuring that both knees are bent at a right angle with your feet facing away from each other. Extend your hips as though you are bringing yourself to a standing position and then bring your left foot to the front again. Planted to the ground so that the knee is at a right angle. Then turn the hind leg so that it points directly behind you as you finish in a lunge position, reverse the whole motion as you come down to a lying position on the ground. Ten Kettlebell Hailo, one of the things that are important to note is that as you brace your body in the correct orientation while you change the position of the kettlebell, it is important that you stay alert and comfortable, move the kettlebell in a circular motion around the body to form something like a halo.

This will strengthen the corps and prepare you for more rigorous exercises down the line. It also plays a critical role in exposing weaknesses as well as a lack of balance. If you are not able to hand off the kettle bells behind you, there is a high chance you will not be able to reach your butt as well. Therefore, if you are going to do the most basic shoulder , it is advisable that you stand with both your feet so that they are in between hip and shoulder width apart. Hold the kettle bells upside down by the horns such that the bell faces upwards, then Rucha feet to the ground as you draw the ribs down. Begin to move the cattle bells around your head while ensuring that you keep an upright posture by not bending the torso in any direction.

Now start moving slowly to avoid hitting your head and make full circles while alternating the orientation. Eleven kettlebell clean, this is a very important exercise that targets the back, the glutes and the hamstrings begin this exercise with the kettlebell on the floor, ensure that it is positioned slightly in front of you in such a way that it lies between your legs and that a shoulder width apart. Now, slightly, bend your knees and hinge at the hips as you grasp the kettlebell, then pull it back in between your legs using one hand such that the thumb points backwards. This creates momentum.

Start driving your hips forward and keep your back as straight as possible. This will help in initiating the upward movement of the kettle bells. Once the kettle bell goes above the height of your belly button, pull it back gently so that you can chapter your fist around and under the bell it will nestle softly at the back of your wrist. And this is referred to as the rack position. Finally push the kettlebell out and allow it to swing down in between your legs, repeat the whole process for three repetitions if you are a beginner, it is important to note that this exercise is even handed. This means that you have to do equal amounts of repetitions on both sides to avoid developing injuries and imbalances.

If you are new to this exercise, you will realize that it is more overpowering than the clean, which essentially causes the bell to flip over and cause a bang on the wrist. Rather than opening your hand, it is advisable that you focus so that you get it around the bell to avoid causing it to flip, so that you can efficiently get the weight to the rack position without any pain. Ensure that your trajectory is straight. Therefore, do not swing the kettlebell to the right or left, instead swing the kettlebell up and pull the bell up and back towards you. Allow your lower body to perform most of the work in getting the bell in its rightful place.

Twelve kettlebell pistols squat. When doing kettlebell exercises, there is so much demand placed on the knee hips and ankle mobility while also requiring that they maintain stability during lifting, considering that the pistol is purely a unilateral exercise of the legs. There is a high chance that any gap in movement is taken into account. Leading you to your weakness is. This means that you have to master the pistol by training your weak points so that you stay safe, strong and perform better at deadlifting, sprinting, cleaning and squatting. In short, all these translate to your overall performance. One of the greatest benefits of learning, the pistol squad is boosting the mobility of the ankle.

This is the movement that comes about when you pull your toes in the direction of your knees, when you have better dorsal flexion, the tibia and the knee move toward over the toes without necessarily causing the knees to rise above the ground. To do this exercise, start by picking up the kettlebell, using both your hands, hold it against your chest, but slightly below your neck region. Now move one leg and then hold it off the ground with the other leg. Start to squat down as you bend one knee while you squat down, hold the kettlebell at the front of your chest and maintain that position when you get closer to the floor. Use the force from your heel to push yourself back up so that you return to the standing position. Repeat this exercise for about three to five reps if you are a beginner.

13 kettlebell jerk, this is another overhead ballistic kettlebell lift that utilizes more leg power and less strength on the upper parts of your body compared to a push press. In other words, the kettlebell jerk is a powerful lift that allows one to perform as many reps as possible. You can even get a heavier weight overhead when performing the kettlebell jerk than when doing a kettlebell push press. It also plays a central role in giving you more cardiorespiratory training. Therefore, in addition to the benefits that you get from the Bush press, the jerk helps you to lower the stress levels on your shoulder joints by simply

engaging more leg power. It needs more stability on the shoulders for the sake of fixation, and therefore it has the potential to create incredibly stable shoulders.

As mentioned, it uses lower leg power and this helps in developing power around the calves, which in turn increases the ankle joint stability. Before you can attempt the jerk, it is important that you master the overhead press and the push press first. This is because it will offer you the opportunity to perfectly get the bell path, train the body, to fixate the kettlebell correctly and practice the dip in a very simple lift. All these techniques are very important when learning the technique for you to get into the very first dip with your heels, the mobility of the ankles is key. To catch the cattle, the bell is a quarter overhead squat position.

It is essential that you comfortably get into position with vertical arms. This is because the exercise is more demanding on the mobility of your upper back, lower back and the shoulders as compared to the overhead lock out position. The best test is for you to try doing broomstick overhead squats. If you cannot get to a quarter squat position with vertical arms, then you have lots of mobility work to do before you can perform the kettlebell jerk. Once you have everything ready, start by holding the kettlebell by the handle, calling the kettlebell to your shoulders, by simply extending your hips and legs as you pull it towards the shoulders. As you do so, ensure that you are rotating your wrist such that your palm faces forward and this will serve as your starting position.

Now begin to dip your body slightly, bending the knees while maintaining the torso in an upright posture. Immediately start reversing the direction as you drive through your heels. In other words, you should jump to create momentum. As you do that, press the kettlebell overhead to lockout by extending your arms, using the momentum of your body to move the weight. Then receive the weight overhead by returning to a squat position under the weight and keep the weight overhead before you can return to a standing position. Lower the weight and repeat the whole process for about three to five reps if you are a beginner.

Kettlebell Workout Plans

In this chapter, we'll discuss beginners intermediate and advanced level kettlebell workout plans. Just as we mentioned earlier, it is critical that you engage in kettlebell exercises that your body can handle, this means that if you are just getting started as a beginner, you are not supposed to engage in high intensity kettlebell workouts. Here we have three levels that will help guide how you engage in exercises that are suitable for your strength and level of flexibility to avoid unnecessary injuries. Beginner level workouts, the main objective of this is to increase your muscular strength as well as endurance in a large number of muscles in the body. It also plays a significant role in boosting the performance of your cardiovascular system.

The total time recommended lies between 15 and 45 minutes. Additionally, the total number of circuits to be performed in a single workout should be three. This is laid out in the table below. Kettlebell, swing, one to three minutes. One thing you have to remember here is to drive your hip forward smoothly, but with energy as you swing the kettlebell forward. Kettlebell goblet half gets up one to three minutes. Here it is critical that you squat as low as you possibly can and then try to drive your hips back up through your heels. Kettlebell one arm row one to three minutes with this exercise, it is essential that you pull the kettlebell toward your tummy while ensuring that your spine maintains a straight posture.

That is the back straight and the chest out. Then keep your elbows tucked in one arm overhead. Press one to three minutes. This is a great alternative to the common bench press we are familiar with. However, with the overhead press, it demands a compound, wrist and movement of the arms. Kettlebell Halo one to three minutes as you exercise, one thing you have to bear in mind is to keep your lower back in its natural arch and to pivot. Intermediate level kettlebell workouts, the main objective of this level of workout is to increase muscular strength and endurance. It is more rigorous than the beginner level and can work the muscles three times as much. It also plays a critical role in boosting the performance of the cardiovascular system.

The total amount of time taken here is estimated at 40 minutes, the total number of circuits to be performed at this level is three. Kettlebell, swing, 12 to 15 minutes here, it is important that your glutes and hips drive the kettlebell forward instead of using your arms. The trick is to ensure that both the hips and the glutes are engaged throughout the exercise. One arm kettlebell floor press, eight to 10 repetitions per side, always remember to turn your wrist towards the feet while pressing the kettlebell in the upward direction, kettlebell Turkish, get up six to eight repetitions per side. This is quite a complex exercise that features a couple of movements. The most critical movement in this case is sliding the leg up in front of you so that it can offer you the support that you need while in a lunge position.

Kettlebell goblets, squat 12 to 15 minutes, get as low as possible without allowing your tailbone to tuck under your butt.

Advanced level kettlebell workouts, the advanced level of kettlebell workouts is suitable for those that have gone through the first two levels we have discussed and have attained a strong level of flexibility and muscular strength enough to handle the advanced workouts. This level does not only promote muscular strength and endurance, but it also pays closer attention to strengthening the core and boosting the cardio capacity. The recommended length of time engaging in this level per chapter is 40 minutes, while the total number of circuits to be performed per workout is three.

Kettlebell windmill eight to 10 repetitions per side, because this is a challenging exercise, it is advisable that you start with a lightweight kettlebell. At first, when you raise the kettlebell overhead, it is critical that you keep your eyes fixated on the weight so that you maintain proper shoulder alignment. Kettlebell deadlift, aim for at least 15 repetitions here. It is important that you engage the core, tighten the glutes and keep your arms as straight as possible when raising the body. The best way to achieve this is to ensure that you push up through your feet. Do not try to pull the kettlebell using your arms. Instead, allow it to come naturally with you as you bring your body to a standing position. Kettlebell clean 15 to 18 repetitions while doing the kettlebell clean.

Remember that the grip position is important as you begin to ensure that you keep your knees bent, as you reach down to grip the handle of the kettlebell using your right hand. It is also important that you keep your thumb behind you while in Iraq. The kettlebell should rest on your forearm, tucked closer to your body while your fist is held at the chest level. Kettlebell split Gerke four to five per leg at first and gradually build it up to eight to 10 as your fitness level increases. If you are going to do this right, it is advisable that you master the clean and the overhead press first, which form the most critical stages of this complex workout kettlebell, pistil, squat four to five per at first and gradually build it up to eight to 10 as your fitness level increases when going up to a standing position, ensure that you drive up using your heels.

Kettlebell Workout Tips & Tricks

In this chapter, we'll discover tips and tricks to use when performing kettlebell workouts. Tips you need to perform the kettlebell swing for you to perform the kettlebell swing. We have discussed it above. It is critical that you maintain the right posture as much as you can, even though it's hard. Some of these tips will help you do it right. Load the heels and not your toes. Try as much as you can to maintain a flat back throughout the exercise. Ensure that you keep your shoulders in their sockets when lifting your chest. Try not to hinge your lower back, take in deep and soft breaths when going up and breathe out nice and soft when coming down. Stand tall throughout the exercise while squeezing your abs.

Tips on how to perfect the single leg deadlift, these include maintaining a tight grip while you keep the shoulder and your back aligned throughout the exercise. Ensure that you maintain the weight on the heel. Instigate movements by simply moving one of your feet towards the back. It is important that you try hard not to arch your lower back. Come down slowly while maintaining control so that you do not rotate your hind leg lest you trip and fall. And share your movements, go as far as you are comfortable without necessarily going beyond your limit of stability and flexibility.

Recap

Indeed, kettlebells have come a very long way from the time when they were used as muscle building tools for strong men in Russia today they are used as fitness tools by both men and women around the world. They are no longer just for building strength, but also endurance, power and weight loss. Therefore, instead of investing lots of money, buying a treadmill, you can choose to lose weight with simple kettle bells that are quite inexpensive. One thing that is important to note is that training with kettlebells is very advantageous. This is because you will not only enable you to meet your fitness goals, but also adopt a healthier lifestyle that protects you against a wide range of dangerous medical conditions.

If you are looking for a fitness workout that is challenging enough and has a proven track record of benefits, kettlebell boot camp is the one for you. They are not only inherently strength based, but also have the ability to challenge the muscles because all you are doing is lifting weights but working a wide range of major muscles across the body. The more weight you add, the stronger you become. The good news with kettlebells is that you can use them for cardio, too, because most kettlebell exercises involve hundreds of both major and minor muscles and joints in the body. It requires a great deal of energy, and this means that the heart and the lungs have to be working very well to achieve this.

The kettlebell workouts are programmed in some sort of circuit, they will promote both strength and cardio performance simultaneously. It is because of this, that kettlebell training is gaining popularity as a tool that also saves time while generating more results. If you are a kettlebell workout beginner, one thing that you have to bear in mind is getting proper instructions from someone who is certified. Most beginners think they can do this alone at home without a trainer. However, if you lift weights without the proper form, you risk causing injuries. The main reason is also that most of the kettlebell exercises we have discussed in this training manual are complex and require practice and guidance from a certified expert trainer.

Once you have learned the kettlebell moves while using lightweights, you will begin to gain muscular strength, flexibility and endurance and soon you can proceed to heavier weights, the more you can make your workouts to be challenging, as long as the body can handle it, the more calories you will burn and the more weight you will lose. If you realize that you are losing your form, feeling faint pain or dizzy, it is critical that you stop exercising immediately. If you are suffering from any medical conditions, always ensure that you consult with your doctor before you can start kettlebell training. Also, notify your trainer of your medical conditions or injuries so that they can modify certain exercises to suit you and avoid further injuries. So what are you still waiting for? Get down to it and get back in shape.

Mindset Conditioning

In this chapter, we'll talk about the importance of mindset conditioning in gaining muscles, roadblocks, brick walls, obstacles, bumps in the road reasons or whatever you call them, they exist and they get in your way daily in our quest to be healthy and fit. Stop giving excuses. Remember that you can have results or excuses, not both. Never let excuses hinder your quest for a healthier and happier life. Also, due to the present access to higher caloric food, the fitness excuses that once ensure our survival now send us to an early grave. The best way to get back on board is to stop making excuses. Now let's talk about the five most common fitness excuses people use to avoid exercising. I don't have enough time. I have no motivation to workout.

I feel intimidated by the fit people there. I don't have anyone to train with. The gym is too expensive or far. These are some of the standard excuses for not making it to the gym that can be heard around the office, school or park every day. To achieve your health and fitness goals, you have to stop making excuses. But not just that. Your mindset plays a significant role as well. A positive mindset is the most powerful tool for reaching your goals. The way you perceive your fitness journey will either make or break your goals. Next, we'll talk about the power of mindset. Why mindset? Because fitness begins with the mind, not the body. The mind has always been at the core of building muscle.

Before you begin counting your muscle mass, the first step to building lean muscle is to get your mindset right. The essentiality of having a strong mind is often overshadowed by being strong physically. If your mindset is right, you will have mental willpower and direction towards your goal, which sets you up for success. One major mistake far too many people make is failing to adopt the right mindset and then falling off the bandwagon before they really even get started. Now, let's talk about the five simple techniques that can help you mentally prepare yourself to learn the fastest way to gain lean mass and ensure you're on the way to achieving your dream body. No one sets specific and achievable goals. No, to cultivate patience.

Number three, hard work is your only shortcut number for every one is different. Don't compare number five, be completely committed. No one sets specific and achievable goals. Now, let's be honest, ask yourself, how much muscle do you want to gain? 10 pounds, 20 pounds? You need to be specific. Don't just estimate or simply see how it goes, because this is going to be the important factor that helps hold you accountable to follow through on your plans and ensure results. People who don't outline exactly what they're aiming to achieve often end up struggling for the right direction, for their muscle gain diet plan in conjunction with their workout plan.

Make your goals specific. Write them down posted on your mirror, your bedroom wall, set your phone screen, just anything that you will see every day. Mindset conditioning has immense power in fueling your determination and commitment in your goal to ultimate successful muscle gain.

No, to cultivate patience upon setting your specific goal, it's time to practice and cultivate patience. Muscle gain isn't going to happen overnight. If you're not ready and prepared for a long journey, you're bound to drop out from the game in no time. So many people expect results in a minimal time frame and then lose interest when their desired muscle gain is nowhere to be seen. Most athletes can build about one to three pounds of muscle per month, Of course, highly depending on their diet and how hard they're working for their muscle gain.

So if you're expecting to gain ten pounds by next month, you're going to be disappointed. Nothing comes easily. Eat smart, work hard and most importantly, have the patience for results. If you're working with the right muscle game plan, eventually the results will prove to you all it's worth. Number three, hard work is your only shortcut. There really isn't any shortcut to muscle gaining. The only way to gain muscle is to invest hard work into building and maintaining it. If you're someone who's always looking for the latest quick fix that confidently promises rapid results with little to no effort, you will be greatly disappointed.

A good diet designed for muscle gain and at the same time incorporated with constant effort in the gym with the correct workout is the only way to get you the progress and results you're after. There is no other way. The sooner you can accept this fact and be prepared or get started, the sooner and more achievable your goal toward muscle gain is going to come true. Number for every one is different. Do not compare yourself to others. The ways that your body absorbs nutrients and reacts towards workouts you do are different from other people.

Everyone's body is unique and different. Another person might build muscle at a certain rate, but that doesn't necessarily mean that you will do unnecessary comparisons that bring disappointment and zero help towards your goal. Focus on your own body, aim for your goals, your plan, your results.

And all you should think of is how to progress until you achieve your dream body mass. Remember, nobody else has your body. You do focus only on yourself. Number five, be completely committed, improve your muscle, gaining mindset by mentally preparing yourself to be completely committed in this process. For instance, commit yourself one hundred percent for at least six months, if not more, set short term, achievable goals, a significant amount of muscle you wish to build and it'll keep you on track working towards those goals. This mindset helps you to be realistic.

You won't expect immediate results, but instead you'll be focusing on the process and duration because you understand and are aware that muscle gaining takes time and effort. When you are mentally prepared to commit over a time frame, you will persevere through the process. Here's some key motivational strategies you can use to keep you in the Book. When things get tough, journaling helps you keep track of your progress. Taking progress pictures is super satisfying as you watch your body evolve each day. Having a workout or diet support, buddy or partner, mental and physical support play a big role in helping you stay motivated.

Muscle Building Diet

In this chapter, we'll talk about muscle pumping diets, high protein diets such as Zone, Atkins and Sugar Busters have come and gone for decades, their popularity rising and falling like waves in the ocean. While high protein diets do usually lead to weight loss, they may be unbalanced meal plans that sometimes restrict entire food groups and fail to meet humans essential needs for vitamins, minerals and fiber. However, that doesn't have to be the case. Several studies comparing high protein, low carbohydrate diets with high carbohydrate, low protein diets found high protein diets to be just as effective and sometimes even more effective. Did you know that protein is one of the nutrients, along with carbohydrate, fat, vitamins, minerals and water? The source of all of these nutrients is good.

Some food contains much higher amounts of specific nutrients than others, and sometimes we refer to certain foods as protein food. It's important to realize that all food contains more than one nutrient and most food contains substantial amounts of several nutrients. For example, meat, which is a good source of protein, carbohydrates, fat, riboflavin and calcium protein is an essential nutrient. There is no life without protein. Protein is contained in every part of your body: the skin, hair, blood, body, organs, eyes, even fingernails and bone. So why exactly is protein so important? Protein has a critical physiological function.

It is primarily used in the body to build, maintain and repair body tissues in the event that protein intake is greater than that required by the body. For this primary function, excessive protein is converted to energy for immediate use or stored in the body is fat protein. Energy will be used only after other energy sources. Carbohydrates and fat are exhausted or unavailable. Protein is available from both animal and plant sources. The typical U.S. diet is a mixture of protein sources. Variety and choices will provide an adequate diet. The following are some examples of protein content. In some typical food, three ounces of chicken contains 20 grams of protein. Three ounces of ground beef contains 21 grams of protein.

Two ounces of pork chop contains 15 grams of protein. Three quarters of a cup of beans contains 11 grams of protein. Two tablespoons of peanut butter contains eight grams of protein. One half cup of soybeans contains 10 grams of protein. And if you're wondering about the protein serving size, here's some references. One ounce of meat is equal to the size of a matchbox. Three ounces of meat is equal to the size of a deck of cards. One ounce of cheese is equal to the size of four dice or one slice. Two tablespoons of nut butter is equal to the size of a ping pong ball. The amount of protein needed varies for different age groups, size and growth stages.

Even though an adult has achieved maximum growth, protein is required for maintaining body tissues. Periods of growth, including infancy, childhood and pregnancy, increased the protein needed to provide building materials. Physiological states such as injury, surgery or burns increase the need for protein to provide repairing materials. Surveys have shown that Americans eat almost twice as much protein as their bodies need. This is probably because of ample supplies of high quality protein and a preference for meat and other animal sources of protein. Food consumption. Surveys show an average protein intake of approximately 100 grams per day. About 70 percent of the protein is from animal products.

The total protein intake supplies. Twelve percent of the total calories. Even with average intakes which are high, some segments of our population may have marginal protein intakes, including low income elderly and pregnant and lactating women. In less developed countries, the protein deficiency disease kwashiorkor is seen in growing children. Now let's talk about protein powder. It has become a popular protein source for people trying to improve athletic performance and build muscle mass for people with cancer. They can provide necessary protein to their diet and help maintain muscle tissue during treatments when experiencing a lack of appetite for eating meats or other high protein foods.

Avoid protein powder that contains other ingredients such as creatine, vitamins or minerals. While these may be high in protein, they tend to be low in calories, so adding higher calorie additions can be beneficial. Did you know that way? Protein concentrate is very common and the most affordable form of whey protein. It does contain some lactose whey protein isolate is a more concentrated form of whey protein, with little to no fat or lactose. It's an acceptable protein source for people on a lactose restricted diet or with lactose intolerance. Hemp protein is a near complete plant.

Vegan protein that offers the inflammation fighting power of omega three essential fatty acids and is high in fiber, protein powder is a plant based protein vegan and highly digestible. It has a fluffy texture. Soy protein powder comes in either soy protein isolate or soy protein concentrate compared to dairy based protein powders. Soy protein powders do not dissolve as well, may have a Beeny taste and can cause gas for people sensitive to soy sugars. Furthermore, there are so many ways that you can add more protein into your diet cheese, melt your cheese on sandwiches, breads, tortillas, hamburgers, hot dogs, other meats or fish, vegetables, eggs or desserts such as stewed fruits or pies.

Or you can grade it and add it to soups, sauces, casseroles, vegetable dishes, mashed potatoes, rice, noodles or meatloaf, cottage cheese or ricotta cheese mix with or use with fruits and vegetables. Add them to casseroles, spaghetti, noodles and egg dishes such as omelets, scrambled eggs and souffles, milk or soy milk in beverages, cooking hot cereals, soups, cocas and puddings in place of water, and dried milk powder. You can choose to add this to regular milk and milk drinks, such as pasteurized eggnog and milkshakes, or used in casseroles, meatloaf, breads, muffins, sauces or any milk based dessert yogurt. Add yogurt to cereals, fruits, gelatin and pies.

Or you can use a blender whip with soft or cooked fruits. You can even sandwich ice cream or frozen yogurt between pound cake cookies or graham crackers. Eggs add chopped hard cooked eggs to salads and dressings, vegetables, casseroles and meat salads. Add extra eggs or egg whites to quiches, pancakes and French toast. Add extra egg whites to scrambled eggs and omelets. Egg whites are a great way to add more protein without saturated fat or cholesterol nuts, seeds, wheat, germs and oats. In fact, there are several ways to add them into your diet. You can sprinkle them on fruit, cereal, ice cream, yogurt, vegetables, salads and toast as a crunchy topping. Or you can blend them with parsley, spinach, herbs and cream for a noodle, pasta or vegetable sauce.

Meat and fish. Add chopped cooked meat and fish to vegetables, salads, casseroles, soups or sauces. You can use them as an omelet, sandwich fillings and chicken stuffing. We all know that a high protein diet is good for muscle building. However, please do not take excessive protein. Excessive intake of protein will lead you to certain health risks. Some of the examples of health risks include ketosis, colorectal cancer, heart disease and kidney disease. In addition, there are certain types of protein that you need to take note of. Although research has shown that high protein diets produce positive effects on blood glucose and blood lipid levels by decreasing circulating insulin, reducing triglycerides and raising HDL levels, there is minimal effect on LDL levels. It's important to remember that even with an emphasis on lean protein, this type of diet is still higher in total fat, saturated fat and cholesterol and lower protein.

High carbohydrate diets and long term effects remain unknown. Red meat high protein diets tend to be heavy on red meat, even though data is inconclusive. High intakes of both red meat and processed meats, particularly if cooked at high temperatures, have been linked to an increased risk of diverticulitis in men. Calcium. Since high protein diets are directly related to a higher output of urinary calcium. Researchers in the 1990s concluded that high protein intakes had an adverse effect on bones. We now know that's not the case. If accompanied by adequate calcium, about three servings of low fat dairy per day or the equivalent high protein diets can not only increase calcium uptake absorbing as much as 25 percent, but also enhance bone health, preserving bone even during weight loss, according to a 2008 Journal of Nutrition study.

Muscle Boosting Supplements

In this chapter, we'll talk about the must have muscle gaining supplements. Yes, you can definitely build muscles without taking supplements, but this will take a much longer period of time to achieve the same results as those who took the right supplements. So ask yourself, do you want to shave off months of unnecessary hard work and get results fast? If your answer is yes, then you should invest in supplements. Without further ado, let's get started generally to build up muscle. It's still better to achieve it through diet and exercise. While supplementation should only be used for additive effects, nonetheless, it shouldn't be pushed aside as supplements are still generally used for health and building muscle foods are usually insufficient for anyone that's looking to gain muscle in the fastest manner.

The best option is to take in the right supplements that your body needs. The top three most used supplements are creatine, vitamin D and Omega three supplements from fish oil. You might wonder if omega three fatty acids from flexor chia seeds should be considered as well. But the fact is Flaxton chia seeds don't provide sufficient supplement on their own flax. And she has. Seeds are found in the form of alpha linoleic acid, which has to be converted by the body into usable form. And the ratio conversion is rather poor. Number one, creatine. Creatine is a molecule produced in the body where it stores high energy phosphate groups in the form of phosphate, creatine or creatine.

Phosphate creatine supplementation confers a variety of health risks, notably neuroprotective and cardio protective. It's usually used by athletes to increase both power output and lean mass. There are various types of creatine and creatine. Manoah hydrate is the most affordable and most effective. It dissolves in water more easily and is best to be taken five grams a day daily while consuming it like any other vitamin. Higher doses up to 10 grams a day may be prudent for those with a high amount of muscle mass and high activity levels. Stomach cramping can occur when creatinine is supplemented without sufficient water. Diarrhea and nausea can occur when too much creatine is supplemented at once, in which case doses should be spread out over the day and taken with meals. No.

Two, Vitamin D is a fat soluble nutrient, and it is one of the 24 micronutrients critical for human survival. The sun is the major natural source of the nutrient, but vitamin D is also found naturally in fish and eggs. While it is also present in dairy products, supplemental vitamin D is associated with a wide range of benefits, including increased cognition, immune health, bone health and wellbeing, while reducing the risk of cancer, heart disease, diabetes and multiple sclerosis. People deficient in vitamin D may also experience increased testosterone levels after supplementation, which can be remedied where the body produces vitamin D from cholesterol. Provided there is an adequate amount of UV light from sun exposure.

Most people are not deficient in vitamin D, but they don't have an optimal level of vitamin D either. Due to the many health benefits of vitamin D, supplementation is encouraged if optimal levels are not present in the body. The recommended daily allowance for vitamin D is currently set at 400 to 800 international units a day. But this is too low for adults. The safe upper limit in the United States in Canada is 4000 IU a day. But research suggests that the true safe upper limit is ten thousand IU a day. As Vitamin D is fat soluble, it has to be taken with a fatty acid that can serve as a transport and it should be taken daily with meals or a source of fat like fish oil. It's best to be taken earlier in the day as it may disrupt sleep patterns if taken later in the evening.

Before we proceed to the third top supplement, let me share with you some supplement facts. Vitamin D, vitamin D deficiency is relatively common in athletes and is associated with muscle weakness and atrophy, specifically type two, muscle fiber atrophy. Skipping out on this vitamin is just as bad as skipping out on day number three, omega three fish oil fish oils. The common term used to refer to two kinds of omega three fatty acids, expensive acid and docos to Novik acid. And they're usually found in fish animal products as well as phytoplankton. Fish oil is recommended as a source of these omega three fatty acids as it's the cheapest and most common source of them.

Fish oil provides a variety of benefits when supplemented, particularly when the ratio of omega three and omega six fatty acids in the body is almost equal or one to one. Did you know that the average diet, red meat, eggs and so forth is high in omega six fatty acids, which is why fish oil is recommended to balance the ratio. A ratio of roughly one to one is associated with healthier blood vessels, a lower lipid count and a reduced risk for plaque buildup. Moreover, fish oil can decrease the risk of diabetes in several forms of cancer, including breast cancer.

Fish oil works primarily through Icaza NEUTZE, which are signaling molecules and a proper ratio of omega three to six fatty acids will influence which Icaza leads are released in response to stress. It should be noted that fish oil can also reduce triglycerides in people with high triglyceride levels. However, it can also increase cholesterol, so care should be taken before supplementing fish oil. For this purpose, fish oil doses vary depending on the goal of supplementation. As for general health, 250 milligrams of combined EPA and DHEA is the minimum dose and can be obtained via fish intake. Supplement fact's fish oil can reduce blood clotting and should be supplemented with caution if blood thinning medications, aspirin, warfarin or clopidogrel are already present in the body.

Next, we'll talk about lists of foods and supplements to avoid when it comes to determining what food you should and should not eat. The only significant point is that calories matter more than specific foods. Adequate macro and micro nutrition are an essential part of a healthy diet, and nonetheless, proper caloric intake is the most important rule, regardless of the source. And whether or not the food is naturally clean or dirty, preparation is the key to eating healthy. It may sound tricky and complex to prepare. Don't overthink it. Instead, choose food that you enjoy eating and make a balanced meal.

Various nutrition studies have indicated that having excess body fat type two diabetes and increase in weight are resulting from consuming and storing excess calories than one burns.

Eating too much of any type of calories, whether from Whole Foods or not, will cause these problems. Generally, the food that you really need to avoid when bulking is junk food and sugary food sugars are the main factors that you really need to look out for. Is there present in foods particularly that aren't fresh, frozen or dried? Additionally, sources such as pasta sauce, ketchup and chili sauce contain sugar as well. You should also avoid fruit juices and fizzy drinks.

There's various sugar content that you need to look out for as well. And this list below is generally what you need to keep an eye out for. Muscle development supplements, including testosterone booster and protein supplements, are compounds that act to enhance muscle protein synthesis or otherwise enhance muscle mass. There are various supplements that would improve muscle growth, but only a handful of them are actually scientifically proven to work if consumed in the recommended method. Supplements that do not offer any muscle growth are considered placebo pills and powders, which is merely an implication to your mind that it affects your body.

These supplements only give you the psychological benefit and if you believe it works than any physiological effect. So save yourself from investing in pills and powders that don't work and invest in those that are proven to promote muscle growth. Taking testosterone boosters is a choice. However, it's always a good idea to cycle testosterone boosters as they do have side effects that could be detrimental to your health excessively, and it could lead to undesirable side effects that are associated with prolonged use. There could be adverse side effects on the testicles like atrophy, and it may reduce stimulation over time. If used, too much.

Compounds that act in the hypothalamus can cause symptoms of what people call adrenal fatigue, where the hypothalamus starts to fatigue. There are three prime examples of compounds that have been scientifically proven that don't affect testosterone levels which are tremulous terrestrial Zema and DS's Partick acid tremulous terrestrial simply doesn't have any factors that would increase testosterone levels as well as body composition and improving exercise performance. Zema is a combination of zinc, magnesium and vitamin B6, which is in the same line with tribalistic estrus.

People who are deficient in zinc and magnesium would benefit for their overall health, but not for increasing testosterone levels. The least C.M.A could do is remove. Micronutrient deficiency that is suppressing testosterone production, acid could increase testosterone levels, but the effects are short lived and temporary. To put it in one word, it's unreliable. There are various scientific studies that have been conducted to determine if increasing testosterone levels can help with boosting muscle gains. The results pretty much show that no matter how high you increase your testosterone levels, it wouldn't help boost muscle building compared to consuming proper diet meals and viable supplements consumed for the purpose of increasing dietary protein.

When food is not taken, it's typically seen as a food product or a meal replacement. Protein powders come from various sources such as milk, beef, rice, peas or hemp, typically used in conjunction with a proper diet to increase dietary protein intake. Some specific types of protein are made for certain scenarios, such as casein protein for a slow release protein and we protein for a faster release. Unfortunately, protein supplements don't directly help you accelerate muscle gain, but consuming enough protein could work compared to consuming protein from food. Protein supplements are convenient for easy snacking, and most of the protein supplements are low in carbs as well as fat, which is good for a proper meal plan. Moreover, they're affordable in terms of price per gram of protein.

Building Your Chest & Biceps

In this chapter, I'll share with you the ultimate chess and best biceps sculpting workouts, these muscle groups will give you the vigor you've been looking for and look good in any outfit. So we're going to focus on that today and we'll walk you through how to execute each workout with the perfect form to ensure maximum muscle growth and minimal injury. First, we'll start off with one of the largest muscle groups of the body. Apart from your legs and back the chest muscles, the three most common ultimate chest workouts are standard push ups, alternating one handed pushups and shoulder reduction. Number one, standard push ups begin in the up position. Hand position can vary, but should be at least slightly wider than the shoulders.

Keep your elbows close to your body and lower yourself very slowly. Keep your back straight and do not allow the knees to touch the floor lower to within one to two inches of the floor and pause momentarily, keeping your back straight, slowly raise your body to the up position, inhale while lowering and exhale while raising yourself back to the starting position. By placing your hands wider apart, you'll be able to work more of the outer pectoral muscles. The standard pushup variation is best for beginners to develop overall pectoral muscles.

And if it's too difficult for you, go ahead and do knee push ups, a variation where you place your knees while doing push ups when you can do at least 30 pushups and are ready to move on to the advanced level, you can switch it up with different pushup variations to challenge yourself and engage different parts of your chest to build those full nasty pecs. Want to challenge myself to do something crazy. Try alternating one handed push ups. Here's how you do it. Your feet should be spread as wide apart as is necessary to maintain stability. The supporting hand should be close to the body. As the push up is performed, the chest and knees should not touch the floor and the other arm will be naturally held up and away from the floor.

Another ultimate chest workout that everyone should include into the routine is shoulder reduction, or more commonly known as chest flies. Unlike push ups and bench presses, the chest fly workout engages the chest muscles more because this is purely a bodybuilding workout to sculpt the chest muscles. Whereas bench presses are more of a powerlifting workout and the range of motion of doing a chest fly is a lot wider than presses. So how do you do it? Here's how you do a standard shoulder reduction: feet should be placed comfortably on the floor, making it easy to push against the ground for stability.

A seat belt helps to reduce excess body movement and isolate and exercise the chest muscles. The upper arm should be in line with the shoulders. Begin with the upper arms parallel to the floor and outstretched to the side, midline to the body or behind the midline for a better stretch. Bring the forearms together in a controlled movement. Do not slam the two pads into each other. The arms naturally tend to drop slightly as the forearms are brought together. Allow the forearm pads to return slowly to their starting position. Breathing techniques can vary, but you should either inhale or exhale on each movement.

Many individuals find it easier to exhale on the concentric contraction of bringing in the forearms together and then inhale on the extension contraction of returning to the starting position. Do not squeeze your hand grip because this detracts from the workout of the chest muscles by using extra energy. This is one common variation. Most people like using a cable for adduction or flies. But you can also use dumbbells or even kettlebell as some prefer standing, while some prefer to do it while laying on a bench. You can always switch things up for more variation because variety is the spice of life. You don't want your workout to be a boring routine. So, well, make sure to keep things fun and interesting.

Honestly, the three workouts that I mentioned earlier can really help you grow some awesome pectoral muscles, especially if you're a beginner. A simple routine with four sets of the three workouts can ensure optimal muscle growth because they engage different angles of the muscles. For more advanced lifters, here are some additional chest workouts. One barbell bench press. Two incline bench presses. Three dumbbell bench presses. Four close grip benches. Press presses are more of a power movement and require proper understanding of each movement and should be performed with the right form.

As injuries are very common with précis, the most common reasons for injury and presses are carrying too much weight and improper form of execution. So how do you properly execute chest press movements? Number one, barbell bench press, lie down on the bench and adjust so your eyes are under the bar. Raise your chest up and tuck your shoulder blades down and squeeze them together. Grab the bar with your hands slightly wider than shoulder length apart slightly, arch your lower back and plant your feet on the ground directly under your knees, shoulder width apart. Unwrap the weight by straightening your arms and then moving it horizontally until it's directly over your shoulders. Remember to squeeze your shoulder blades together when you perform bench presses and tuck your elbows in at a 45 degree angle for safety and proper execution.

A lot of guys risk screwing up their elbows and shoulder joints by not following these two simple tips. Also start late and drop your ego in the gym. Ego lifting is a surefire way to the hospital. And if you don't want to suffer from unnecessary pain and injuries, be honest with yourself and pick the weight you can handle. Your only goal is to make progress in your fitness goal and not impress other people in the gym. No. Two Incline bench presses. As mentioned before, the chest muscles are made up of different parts and angles. The common ones are the upper chest and the lower chest, the outer, middle and inner chest.

The upper chest is the least developed part for the majority and you should really focus on this part more as the upper chest provides the illusion of you having fuller and mightier pecs. And the best workout to target the upper chest is the incline bench. Press one load the bar to an appropriate weight for your training to lay on the bench with your feet flat on the ground driving through to your hips. Your back should be arched and your shoulder blades retracted. Three Take a medium pronated grip covering the ring on the bar. Remove the bar from the rack, holding the weight above your chest with your arms extended. This will be your starting position for lowering the bar to the sternum by flexing the elbows, maintain control and do not bounce the bar off your chest. Your lap should stay tight and elbows slightly drawn in five.

After touching your torso with the bar, extend the elbows to return the bar to the starting position. Number three dumbbell bench press. This can be said to be a more advanced level of push ups as it engages the chest more and you're able to make progress with heavier weights. Here's how you do a dumbbell bench press properly. One lies down on a flat bench with the dumbbell in each hand resting on top of your thighs. The palms of your hands will be facing each other, then using your thighs to help raise the dumbbells up, lift the dumbbells one at a time so you can hold them in front of you at shoulder width three one, sit shoulder width, rotate your wrist forward so that the palms of your hands are facing away from you. The dumbbells should be just to the sides of your chest with your upper arm and forearm creating a ninety degree angle.

Be sure to maintain full control of the dumbbells at all times. This will be your starting position for then, as you breathe out, use your chest to push the dumbbells up, lock your arms at the top of the lift and squeeze your chest. Hold for a second and then begin coming down slowly. Tip. Ideally, lowering the weight should take about twice as long as raising it. Five Repeat the movement for the prescribed amount of repetitions of your training program. Number four Close grip bench press. This workout focuses on the inner pecs and triceps. One lies back on a flat bench using a close grip around shoulder width. Lift the bar from the rack and hold it straight over you with your arms locked.

This will be your starting position. Two as you breathe in, come down slowly until you feel the bar on your middle chest tip. Make sure that as opposed to a regular bench press, you keep the elbows close to the torso at all times in order to maximize triceps involvement. Three After a second pause, bring the bar back to the starting position as you breathe out and push the bar using your triceps muscles, lock your arms in the contracted position, hold for a second and then start coming down slowly again. Tip. It should take at least twice as long to go down than to come up to repeat the movement for the prescribed amount of repetitions. Five. When you're done, place the bar back on the rack.

Biceps are the epitome of fitness. Every man and woman deserves to have some awesome biceps. You should really incorporate biceps workouts into your routine to grow these proud muscles. And here are my best biceps. Sculpting workouts. One standing barbell curl to ez bar preacher curl. Three alternate incline dumbbell curls for reverse wrist curl and wrist curl. Five seated Barbell Curl, six Tooele Dumbbell, Hammer, Curl, No. One standing barbell curl, this is the most basic biceps workout that you can see in boasters in magazines. It engages both of your total biceps at the same time, one with your knees slightly bent and your feet about hip width apart. Grasp a barbell with a shoulder width underhand grip to let the bar hang to your knees, keep your abs pulled in and your elbows stationary.

Three without swaying, slowly curl the bar in an arc towards your shoulders as you exhale for a pause at the top of the movement, squeeze your biceps and slightly lower the bar almost to the start. Five Don't lift the bar completely to your shoulders and don't let it touch your thighs at the bottom in order to keep continuous tension on the biceps. No too easy bar preacher curl. This workout engages your inner biceps and brings out the biceps peak one position, the seat height so your armpits are flush against the pad to place your feet forward to help stabilize your body and grasp the easy bar with an underhand grip so your little fingers are higher than your thumbs.

Your palms supernet out three. Slowly raise the bar to shoulder level, pause and squeeze your biceps, then lower the bar to just short of elbow lockout number three alternate incline dumbbell curl. This is my favorite workout. Hands down because this workout is a perfect isolation workout for the biceps without any cheating movements, because the incline position cancels out most of the cheating momentum, increases the range of motion and you can't really carry much weight when you're lying. Incline one set an incline bench to about a 45 degree angle, too, with a dumbbell in each hand and using a neutral grip, palms facing each other. Let your arms hang straight down below your shoulders.

Three: Keep your elbows still slowly. Bring your right hand up, turning your hand as you lift so your palm faces your shoulder to pause and squeeze the biceps at the top, then lower the weight slowly to the start. Five Repeat with your left hand to complete one rep. I recommend doing ten to twelve reps for three to four sets for this exercise to effectively grow your biceps. Number four, reverse wrist curl and wrist curl. This additional workout trains your wrists and forearms, many people ignore this exercise because they don't see the need for it. But do you want to look like a hunk with huge biceps and triceps and arms like twigs? If you want to look good overall and have strong stabilization muscles to move more weights, add these to compulsory forearm workouts into your workout regimen.

One, grasp a straight bar with an overhand grip, hands about 10 inches apart to kneel on the floor along one side of a flat bench. With your forearms on the bench, let your hands and wrists hang over the edge. Three Curl your hands up as high as possible, then lower the weight to the start position to maximize your range of motion. Keep your thumbs on the underside of the bar for four reps, then use an underhand grip with your hands about four inches apart, thumbs under the bar and perform the same movement. Number five seated barbell curl. This is another variation for bicep curls. One load of barbell with 10 to 20 pounds more than you can do for six to eight reps of regular barbell curls to sit on a short back bench or an adjustable bench set to ninety degrees and rest the bar on your thighs. Three with an underhand shoulder width grip. Curl the bar toward your shoulders, keeping your torso perpendicular to the floor.

Don't lean back too slowly. Lower the weight and repeat to keep constant tension on your biceps. Don't let the bar rest on your thighs between reps. Stop it just before it touches your legs. Number six dual dumbbell hammer curl. This is a killer workout for both forearms and biceps. Every biceps workout routine should have hammer curls in there to complete one stand erect, holding a pair of dumbbells by your sides with your palms facing each other to curl both dumbbells toward your shoulders without turning your wrists or letting your elbows move forward. Three Extend your elbows to slowly return to the start. So there you have it. My ultimate chest and biceps sculpting workouts you can add into your workout routine and grow those highly esteemed muscles.

Celebrity Workout

Everyone wants to look like a celebrity, so if you want to look like one, you can simply model them. In this chapter, we'll learn about the celebrity workout, what they did and how they did it. Everything begins with a game plan and a winning mindset. So if you really want to have that beachbody of your favorite celebrity, decide and commit to your workout plan, first and foremost, make sure you have a clear diet plan laid out and you stick to it until the end of your 30, 60 or 90 day plan. Once your diet's all set and you're confident with what you can eat, it's time to put the workout into play. There are various types of workouts you can choose depending on your goals and what you like to do with your personal time.

The most significant point is that you need to seek something that you enjoy doing or really want to do. It's not necessary to determine the type of workout because it's what you feel you need to do. There are various choices. If you think that this type of workout doesn't appeal to you, you can shift into a different workout. Before we begin, I want to make sure that you understand what you can expect from this topic. Everyone is one hundred percent unique. You can't simply expect to look exactly the same as your idol. For example, do you know the differences between high and low bicep insertions? Performing bicep curls will not change your insertions. Muscle insertions affect all muscles on your body and biceps are a simple example to illustrate this point.

When it comes to celebrity workout plans, they are barely an accurate representation of what the individual actually did. Most celebrity workout plans that you could find on the Internet would probably lack a lot of information about the individual's nutrition recovery protocol, prior training, history and so on. Most importantly, everyone's physique is built differently. Same goes for your abs. Some of you might have four pack abs, some six packs, and some even have eight to ten pack abs. The reason they have so many abs is not because they train harder than anyone else, but because they're genetically gifted with it. So instead of relying on using a celebrity's ideal physique as a target to desire to use them as inspiration to stay consistent in your training and diet, genetics play a significant role in how a person's muscles are developed and shaped.

And no amount of workout will change how you're physiologically built. Now that we've set things straight, let's talk about practicing celebrity workouts. Personally, you can still follow your desired celebrity workout plan as a stepping stone to achieve your goals of muscle building. But in terms of diet plan, it's not ideal to straight out follow their diet plans, even if it's out there for people to look up to. Our daily caloric needs are varied from individual to individual. Even if you have the exact same weight and body metabolism, don't expect to gain the same results as what they've achieved.

Nonetheless, let's look into several celebrity workouts that shape into everyone's desired body. Here's Daniel Craig's physique back in James Bond, Casino Royale, famous for his role as the current James Bond w seven agent in the James Bond franchise films, he spends months to tune his body just for that particular role. He partakes in weight training five days a week, followed by light cardio with stretching on the weekends, practicing the ideal diet plan and having a personal trainer and dietician to keep him in line as he wasn't overweight prior to engaging in this workout, he just needed to lose a proper amount of weight and build muscles. Generally, most people would concentrate on one muscle group per day, working it only once a week.

Daniel works on full body circuits, boosting his heart rate and developing muscle and endurance at the same time. Next, I'll show you his workout routine. So take notes. Now let's look at his full body circuit weekdays with light cardio weekends, Mondays, workout power circuit, ten reps per exercise with three sets clean and press weighted knee raise weighted step ups. Pull ups, incline push up tricep dips. Tuesday's workout chest and back 10 reps per exercise with four sets, incline bench press, pull up, incline, push up incline peak flies, Wednesday's workout legs, 10 reps per exercise with four sets squat straight leg deadlift, hamstring curl weighted lunge.

Thursday's workout, shoulders and arms, 10 reps per exercise with four sets, incline bicep curls, tricep dips, lateral raises, shoulder press. Friday's workout power circuit 10 reps per exercise with three sets clean and press weighted knee raise weighted step ups pull up incline push up tricep dips Saturday and Sunday's workout light cardio such as outdoor and physical activities. A full body circuit is a workout that jumps from one exercise to another with minimal rest. This is the optimum way to build muscle and burn fat at the same time.

Moreover, it's a more effective workout in burning fat than a traditional cardio routine.

Hugh Jackman, best known for his long running roles as the Wolverine in the X-Men film series, as well as various lead roles in movies such as Van Helsing, The Prestige and Lamees Rob, which got him nominated for best actor in the Academy Award before he co starred in his role as Wolverine, he worked together with his trainer, David Kingsbury, to get his desired shape for the role as Wolverine. According to his trainer, he was already in good shape before he proceeded to build up his muscle mass and leanness for the role. Due to that, he focused more on direct strength workouts with one to five reps, followed by higher reps schemes with a combination of low intensity training and intervals to keep the body fat levels down while bulking.

The weight training remained more or less the same during the whole process, with the only change in his body fat levels coming from the volume of cardio he was prescribed in the amount of calories consumed. According to his personal trainer, his diet plan was a straightforward plan. By having carbs on weight training days and low carb on normal days in terms of supplement consumption, he took creatine for bulking, while for pre and post workout he took to preserve lean muscle mass and universal carnitine to help metabolize fatty acids to improve strength and size while keeping body fat to a minimum.

Who practices a progressive overload workout to ensure continual strength gains designed on a four week schedule. The reps for the main lifts are changed each week. For the first three weeks, the weight will be increased each week. During the first week, the weight is reduced to be able to perform ten reps instead. The general outlook of the training schedule is as follows. Week one four sets with five reps each week to four sets with four reps each week, three four sets with three reps each week for four sets with ten reps each. Chris Evans, best known for his superhero roles as the Marvel Comics character, Captain America in the Marvel Cinematic Universe and The Human Torch in Fantastic Four.

He gained serious muscle mass with an intensive workout routine in order to play the role as Captain America as portrayed in the comic version. His training was mainly focused on resistance training with only minimal cardio, which is about 20 minutes a day. Generally, this workout is suitable to those who have been training for over six months consecutively and want to shift towards a different workout plan. Resistance training routine, it works on different parts of your body to achieve a balance. Day one, shoulders seated, barbell press lateral raises, dumbbell press seated, rear deltoid raise shrugs, 10 minute HIIT training chapter on treadmill or bike day to chest.

Flat bench press incline chest press, bench flyes decline, chest press push ups on a bosu ball. Day three legs, barbell squats, leg press, , squats, lunges, seated catchphrases, 10 minute HIIT training chapter on treadmill or bike day. Four arms and core. Barbell bicep curls, skull crushers, incline seated bicep curls, cable hammer curls, dips, close grip bench press, ab crunches with legs raised thirty seconds stability ball plank stability ball jackknife oblique crunches on stability ball each side the five back pull ups, seated row lat pulldowns stiff leg barbell deadlift bent over barbell row ten minute HIIT training chapter on treadmill or bike day six and seven rest body and energy recovery to build up muscle mass.

It's recommended to consume whey protein drinks about an hour before and after a workout for muscle recovery and growth. The workout routine focuses on four sets of each exercise and eight to ten repetitions practice four sets of each exercise in a row and take a minute rest between each set and before jumping to the next exercise. For any beginners that would like to start muscle building, the best thing you can do is leverage someone else's knowledge to learn how to workout properly. There are various workout plans that were created by professional fitness specialists, specifically for beginners.

The best way to think of it is that no matter what your desired body looks like, it'll end up in two very simple factors. One having muscle and two having low body fat depending on the body. It's just a matter of the degree of these two factors. While it's impossible to get your ideal body shape that looks exactly like your desired goal, you can get as close as possible simply by aiming to have a similar amount of muscle and a similarly low amount of body fat. So did you have any celebrities who inspired you to get into shape? Go ahead and model them and make it your fitness goal. This is one of the best visualization techniques. Top fitness models and competitors used to be at the top of their game. It's simply because when you see it, you believe it.

Conclusion

In this chapter, we'll discover the secret muscle building techniques for vegans and vegetarians. Did you know that weight loss and weight gain is controlled by the difference between how many calories you take and consume daily? While building muscle, you must eat at a surplus and do resistance training similar to any muscle builder or a person that desires to lose weight. Vegetarians share a similar goal, which is losing fat and building muscle. Now let's talk about some things that may interest you. Number one, building up your muscles is 80 percent from your diet, while the remaining 20 percent comes from your physical exercise and training. Number two, to lose fat and build muscle. You have to eat correctly.

This will be your first and main priority before moving to your physical activities. If you got your diet fixed and in check, you're one step closer to building up muscle. That being said, building muscle as a vegetarian is a daunting task and a complex one due to the fact that you would have a restriction to the certain food you have access to eat. Number three, determining your vegan diet plan is significant to determine what you can and should eat and how you can consume it. Just like any ordinary person that has fixed their diet plan as a vegetarian, it's best to track the calories of everything you eat during the day.

Number four, as a vegetarian, your protein requirements will vary from the usual diet plan that ordinary people practice. You'll probably need to consume a protein supplement with the addition to your personal diet if your strength training. There are various types of protein based food that you can choose from, such as rice, protein, hemp protein and GEMAP protein as well as soy egg or whey protein are viable options, too. If you're not a vegan that avoids foods produced by animals or animal products in any way when it comes to the consumption of vegetable protein, there are various important factors to keep in mind when considering vegetable protein.

There are anti nutritional factors which are commonly found in soy and other vegetable protein isolates that are capable of limiting the extent to which your body's system can utilize the protein. Thus, it is highly important to keep in mind that your body may require a higher consumption of vegetable protein to gain the same effect of a usual consumption of protein. Next, we'll talk about the best vegetable protein powders you could consider one way protein, one of the best choices for vegetarians, especially for muscle builders. Moreover, it helps with cutting down excess weight and supports your health.

Overall, protein can be easily absorbed and digested into your body. Additionally, it's an ideal choice for people who are lactose intolerant as it is tolerable compared to other protein powders. If you're a vegan that's refrained from consuming any dairy products, protein is clearly not your choice as it's derived from cheese production to brown rice protein powder. This is a good option. If you can't opt for whey protein as their gluten and dairy free, they're packed with high levels of antioxidants and nutrients to support weight loss. Three Hemp proteins. This contains a complete amino acid profile. While it's easy to digest and it helps with pre workout it won't cause stomach issues while you're exercising.

Moreover, hemp is a safer plant source of protein in general as it's cultivated using an organic agricultural method. There are various nutrient dense foods that you can gain protein for your plant based diet vegetables such as avocado, broccoli, spinach, sweet potatoes and boiled peas can be your staple vegan. Diet, legumes, especially lentils and beans, which have been the foundation of various diet plans, are plants that you could consider. They are high in protein and dietary fiber. Moreover, they're mainly good food for satiety, balancing blood sugar, maintaining weight and energy. Last but not least, nuts and seeds can be incorporated into your snack or meal diet plan as they offer high amounts of protein, fiber, vitamins and minerals.

There's a saying, if you fail to plan, you're planning to fail. Benjamin Franklin, hence, never underestimate the power of planning out your diet by being self aware with what you can eat and how much you eat daily won. The optimized way to do this is to calculate the calories of everything you consume during the Book of the entire day with the use of a calorie tracking application or a pen and paper. You can check out my fitness pal Dotcom to be used as a calorie tracker to to easily determine how much you should be eating. You need to determine your own total daily energy expenditure or TDE check out one percent Edgecomb if Kalsi, which is a good tool to adjust your calorie intake to match your personal goal, whether that's muscle buildup or fat loss, suffice to say, if you wish to gain muscle, basically you need to eat over your total daily energy expenditure.

If you're losing weight at the same time while building muscles, it's best to remain conservative by staying within five hundred calories above or below respectively. The TDE calculator will only project out the estimated daily caloric needs. Hence, you need to track your daily caloric intake and compare that to your weight loss or gain to determine a more personalized approach. Adjust your daily intake and reassess for the next few weeks. Repeat this step until you're losing weight at the rate determined by your own daily deficit.